With compliments

Knoll AG

experts in wound healing

R.A. Hatz   R. Niedner
W. Vanscheidt   W. Westerhof

Wound Healing and Wound Management

A Guide for Private Practice

Foreword by F.W. Schildberg

With 47 Figures

Springer-Verlag
Berlin Heidelberg New York
London Paris Tokyo
Hong Kong Barcelona
Budapest

Dr. R. A. Hatz
Chirurgische Klinik
Klinikum Großhadern
Marchioninistr. 15
81377 München

Prof. Dr. R. Niedner
Klinikum Ernst von Bergmann
Charlottenstr. 72
14467 Potsdam

Priv.-Doz. Dr. W. Vanscheidt
Universitäts-Hautklinik
Hauptstr. 7
79104 Freiburg i. Br.

Prof. Dr. W. Westerhof
Academic Medical Center
Department of Dermatology
University of Amsterdam
Meibergdreef 9
NL-1105 AZ Amsterdam

Translation by
N. von Jan,
München

Springer-Verlag GmbH & Co KG
Science Communication
Editing Dept. for Medicine
Priv.-Doz. Dr. B. Fruhstorfer, Dr. A. Heinz,
D. Berger, U. Hilpert, K. Kupfer, Heidelberg

ISBN-13:978-3-540-58321-9   e-ISBN-13:978-3-642-79195-6
DOI: 10.1007/978-3-642-79195-6

Layout and Production Supervision: W. Bischoff, Heidelberg
Typesetting: H&S Team für Fotosatz GmbH, Heidelberg

16/3130 – 5 4 3 2 1 0 – Printed on acid-free paper

Foreword

Whenever the integrity of the skin is impaired, via trauma or surgical incision, wounds und wound healing are the natural consequences. Thus, every physician should be interested in the biological processes involved in wound healing. The physician does not usually interfere with these natural processes, knowing that the body heals itself (natura sanat). It is not until the natural wound healing process is disturbed, that we realize how little we know about this area. Our limited knowledge is not even available to most physicians.

Advances in the areas of cell- and molecular biology have also resulted in substantial progress in the field of wound healing. Today, we know that the process of tissue repair occurs in three phases and is controlled by specific cells. These cells release potent mediators which in turn regulate the function of other cells surrounding the area.

"Certain rules apply to the healing of wounds and injured tissue. You must follow nature for nature will never follow you", this sentence writen by Paracelsus in his book "Chirurgia magna" is still valid today. Current reseach in wound healing is exploring these rules and integrating them into new therapeutical concepts. The purpose of this book is to make current knowledge on basic healing processes, research in this area and on wound management available to most physicians.

Due to the importance of wound healing and the successful combination of basic science and clinical aspects, I would like this book to be widely accepted.

Prof. Dr. F.W. Schildberg
Head of the Department of Surgery
Clinic Großhadern
Ludwig-Maximilians-University Munich
Germany

Contents

Abbreviations

bFGF	basic fibroblast growth factor
CAMS	calmodulin
EGF	epidermal growth factor
FGF	fibroblast growth factor
GF	growth factor
GM-CSF	granulocyte-macrophage colony-stimulating factor
ICAM	intercellular adhesion molecule
IFN	interferon
IGF	insulin-like growth factor
IL-1	interleukin-1
IL-2	interleukin-2
IL-6	interleukin-6
IL-8	interleukin-8
PAF	platelet-activating factor
PDGF	platelet-derivating growth factor
PGE_2	prostaglandin E_2
TCDO	tetrachlorodecaoxide
TGF-β	transforming growth factor β
TNF	tumor necrosis factor
VEGF	vascular epidermal growth factor

1 Physiology of Wound Healing

A wound is defined as an interruption of tissue to a greater or lesser extent, which may affect skin, mucosa, or organs. The specific sequence of different processes following wounding has one common aim: repair. This is achieved by very complex and dynamic procedures, in which material is degraded (catabolic phase) and newly synthesized (anabolic phase). Wound healing includes aspects concerning certain cell types, biochemical conditions, localization, and time. In every wound type the healing process runs through three stages, which partly overlap. The first one, the exsudative or inflammatory phase, is followed by the proliferative phase and finally the regenerative phase (Fig. 1).

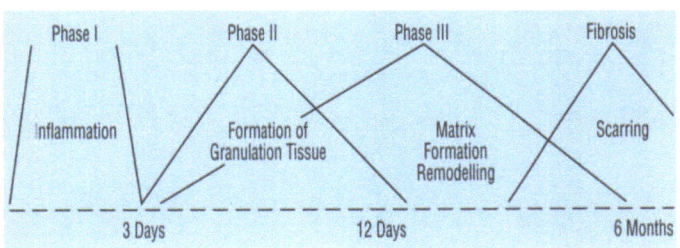

Fig. 1. Phases of wound healing

1.1 Exsudative Phase

Characteristic for the exsudative (or inflammatory) phase – lasting approximately 72 h – is the activation of the blood coagulation system and the release of various mediators from platelets, such as platelet-derived growth factor (PDGF), platelet-activating factor (PAF), thromboxane, serotonine, adrenaline, and complement factors.

Effects of platelets in wound healing

1. Hemostasis
* Aggregation
* Coagulation
2. Secretion of biologically active components
* Vasoactive mediators
* Chemotactic factors
* Growth factors

Fig. 2.
Blood coagulation

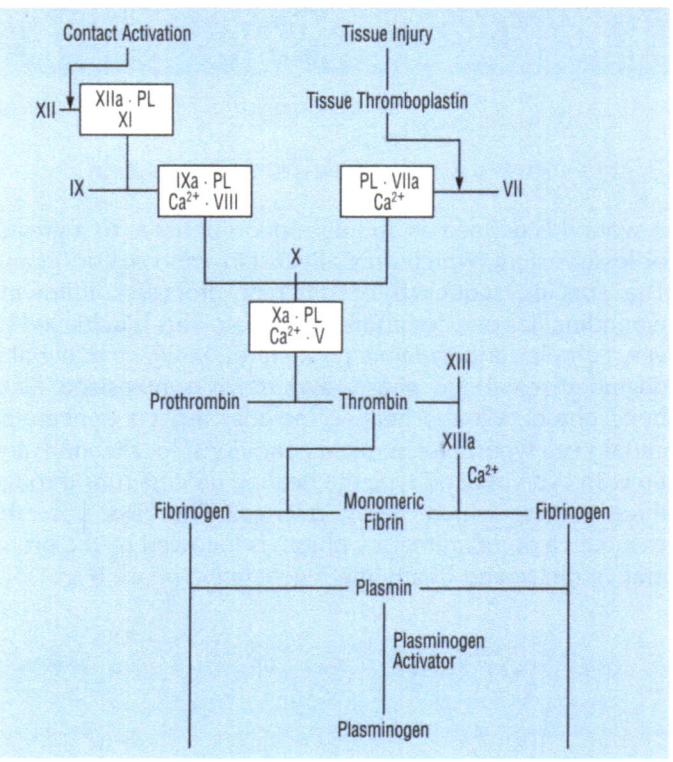

Fig. 3.
Fibrin synthesis

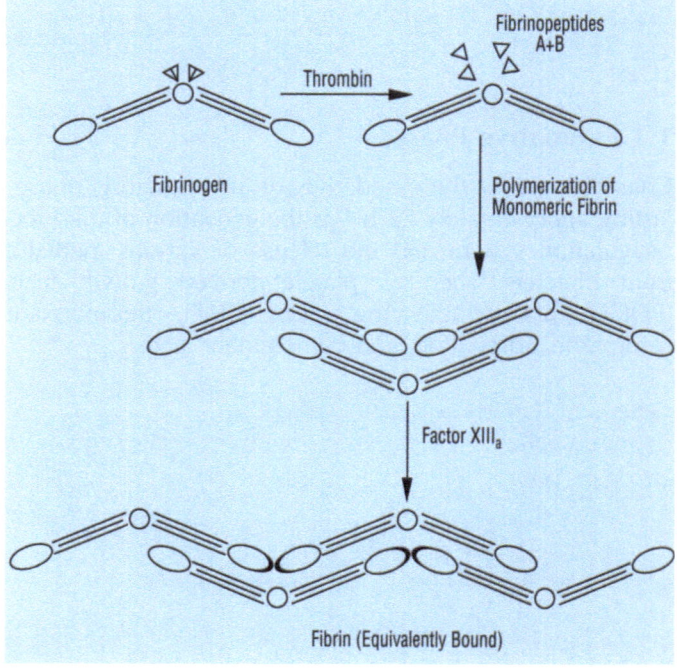

Blood Coagulation

The primary goal of biological repair is the termination of blood loss. Platelets adhere to freshly exposed tissue components, such as collagen and aggregate and by forming a plug lead to coagulation to some extent. Platelets and damaged cells release various mediators activating an entire cascade of factors (Fig. 2) finally transforming fibrin into fibrinogen.

During the final stage of blood coagulation factor XIIIa is produced. By transforming soluble fibrin into its unsoluble form, factor XIIIa stabilizes fibrin (Fig. 3). In addition, it leads to binding of fibronectin to fibroblasts. Monomeric fibrin aggregates form netlike structures, stimulated by active faxtor XIII, constructing the matrix for fibroblast migration. Faxtor XIII is the connecting element between coagulation and cellular processes in wound healing.

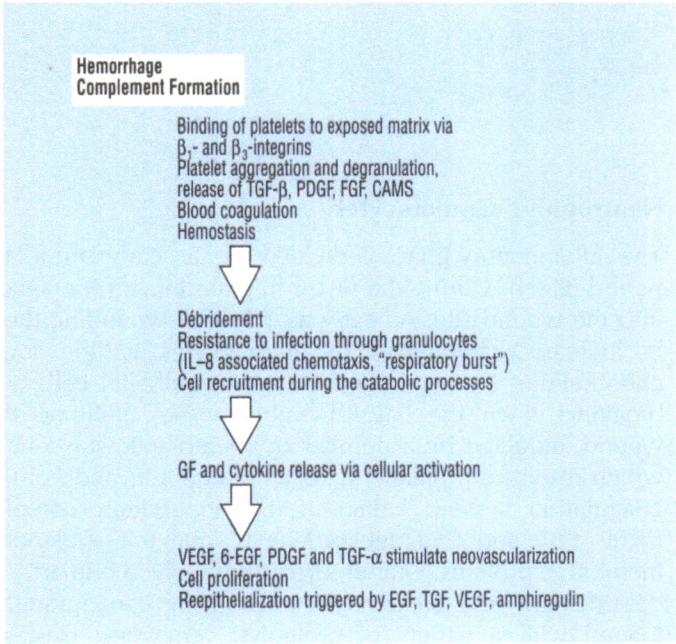

Fig. 4.
Inflammatory mechanisms

To keep blood coagulation and platelet aggregation within a physiological range, the endothelium produces regulatory factors such as prostacyclin (inhibits platelet aggregation), protein C (inactivates coagulation factors V and VIII, inactivates the inhibitor of the t-plasminogen activator through its endothelial cofactor thrombomodulin), and t-plasminogen activator (activates fibrinolysis).

Inflammatory Cells

Within the first phase of wound repair cellular processes are determined by immigrating inflammatory cells (after 2–4 h) and fibroblasts (after 32 h). As satelites of the immune system mostly neutrophilic granulocytes but also macrophages infiltrate the wound. They are attracted by chemotactic substances: complement factors C3a and C5a, degradation products from fibrin and collagen released from blood clots.

Secretory produtcs of granulocytes:

Myeloperoxidase
Elastase
Acidic hydrolase
Neutral proteases
Lysozyme
Lactoferrin
ROS

Neutrophilic Granulocytes

The inflammatory phase is divided into an early and a late period (Fig 4). During the first 6 h, granulocytes immigrate into the wound site. As early as 1 h after wounding there is increased adherence of granulocytes to the local endothelium. By migrating between endothelial cells and breaking down the basal membrane they infiltrate the wound, attracted by a number of chemotactic substances which result from platelet agregation and activation of the coagulation system: kallikrein, fibrinopeptides, complements C3a and C5a, leukotriene B_4 and bacterial outer membrane proteins. Granulocytes are involved primarily in débridement and bacterial defense. They carry granules loaded with a variety of proteolytic enzymes: elastase, acidic hydrolases, lactoferrin, and lysozyme. Lysed granulocytes in combination with wound fluid lead to pus depositon. Therefore, purulent conditions are a quite common observation in wound healing. Granulocytic infiltration comes to an end after a few days if the wound does not become infected with pathogenic bacteria.

Contamination

In infected wounds, granulocytes continuously immigrate, which obviously extends the first phase of repair, leading to marked delay in wound healing (possible abcess formation). Opsonization and phagocytosis are the two most important granulocytic properties during bacterial elimination (Fig. 5).

The surface of the bacterial organism is covered with immunoglobulins and complement C3b (i.e., opsonization), which promotes adherence to and phagocytosis by granulocytes. Known conditions reducing the opsonic capacity of the human immune system are intense catabolic metabolism (e.g., after large operations, trauma), diabetes mellitus, and other diseases. After phagocytosis of the germ

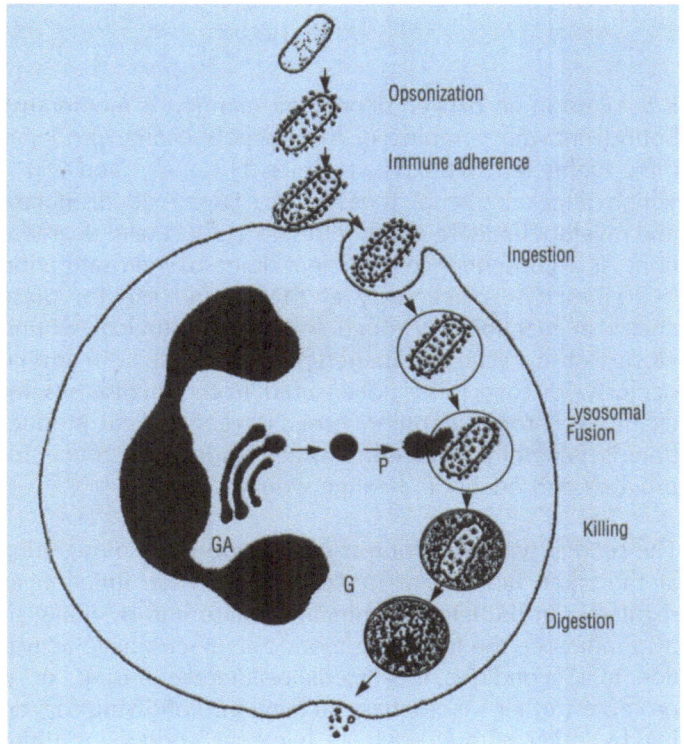

Fig. 5.
Opsonization and phagocytosis.
P, Phagolysosome;
GA, Golgi's
     apparatus;
G, granulocyte

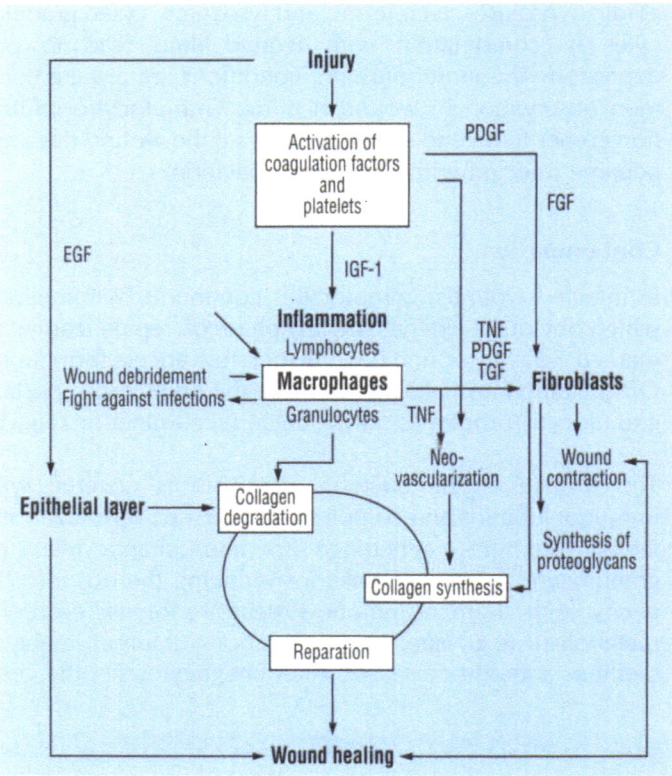

Fig. 5a.
The central role of
macrophages in
wound healing

it is killed in an oxygen-dependent manner: A membrane-bound enzyme complex of the phagolysosome produces three highly reactive oxygenspecies (H_2O_2, O_2^- and OH^-), which attack bacterial membranes. Superoxidedismutase and myeloperoxidase also contribute to successful degradation. As a consequence, sufficient tissue oxygen saturation (> 20 mmHG) is necessary at the wound site for these chemical reactions. Through inadequate surgical wound closure or in a state of impaired perfusion such as in arterial occlusive disease, this is not ensured. In certain diseases, for example, chronic granulomatosis, oxygen radical production is generelly reduced. Oxygen supply is crucial for progress and quality in healing wounds.

The second type of immunocytes in wounds – immigrating at the same time – are macrophages. These function as regulators in the late inflammatory phase and by doing so also influence the following monocyte/macrophage activation. In a second step, local mediators (interferon-α, -β, or -γ) promote further macrophage activation. Following triggering by other stimuli such as bacterial endotoxins (third

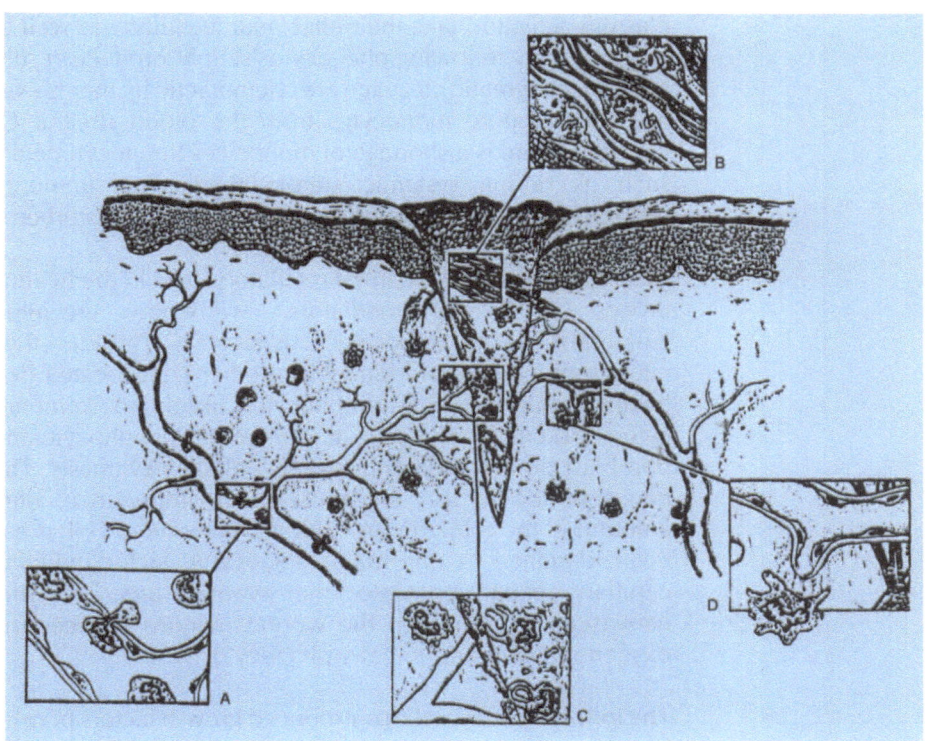

activation step), the wound macrophage is transformed into a cytolytic, phagocytic cell.

Macrophage function in wound healing is necessary for débridement on the one hand, and stimulation and regulation of the repair sequence by secreted cytokines on the other. Some weeks after wounding macrophages are still detectable at the former wound site. As with granulocytes, they produce tissue degrading agents after activation. These proteolytic enzymes (elastase, collagenase, cathepsin B,

Fig. 5b.
The macrophage in wound healing.
A Emigration of blood monocyte into the extra-vascular space.
B Differentiation of monocyte into macrophage.
C Secretion of angiogenetic factor.
D Budding of existing capillary

Steps in eliminating bacterial wound contamination

* Opsonization of bacteria by complement
* Creation of chemotactic factors
* Adhesion of leukocytes to endothelial cells
* Elimination of leukocytes from blood vessels
* Adhesion of opsonized bacteria to polymorphonuclear granulocytes
* Phagocytosis of the bacteria
* Killing and elimination of the bacteria

plasmin activator) take their effect extracellularly as well as intracellularly following phagocytosis. Split products resulting from enzymatic cleavage are chemotactic by themselves and recruit more monocytes from the blood stream. Of course, if there is a shortage of monocytes (monocytopenia) such as during systemic steroid therapy or immunosuppressive therapy, wound healing is severely disturbed.

Macrophages work as central regulatory cells in the healing process. By secreting mediators – well-known are interleukin-1 (IL-1) and tumor necrosis factor α (TNF-α) – they effect proliferation and function of other cells located in a healing wound, such as lymphocytes, fibroblasts, keratinocytes, and endothelial cells. IL-1 increases lymphocyte and fibroblast proliferation and triggers collagen synthesis. The concentration of IL-1 seems to be of importance; high amounts of the cytokine can inhibit proliferation. TNF-α has been identified as one major angiogenic factor inducing capillary expansion into the wound area. Missing neovascularization from the wound margins reduces the oxygen gradient and impairs phagocytosis.

The following macrophage-produced growth factors play an important role in wound healing: basic fibroblast growth factor (bFGF), epidermal growth factor (EGF), PDGF, and transforming growth factor β (TGF-β). These mediators are known as cell growth and cell division promoting and/or inhibiting peptides. Each factor has specific target cells determined by receptors on the cell surface.

Function of activated macrophages

Lysosomal activity, production of complement
γ-Interferon (IFN-γ) production
Thromboplastin secretion
Prostaglandin synthesis
Release of proteases
Phagocytosis
Production of angiogenic factors
Stimulation of fibroblast proliferation and epithelialization
IL-1
TGF-α, -β
TNF-α
FGF
PDGF

Fibroblast growth factor (FGF) has a mitogenic effect on endothelial cells and stimulates fibroblast proliferation. EGF has stimulatory effects on migration and growth of keratinocytes. PDGF is chemotactic and mitogenic for fibroblasts. TGF-β strongly affects chemotaxis of monocytes and macrophages, inhibits proliferation of fibroblasts, T- and B- lymphocytes, and keratinocytes in a reversible manner. Growth factors can work synergistically, but also antagonistically regulating wound healing in a very complex, not fully understood way. Whether growth factors are of therapeutic value in wound healing remains to be clarified.

Overall, macrophages play a prominent role in wound healing processes, and altering their number and function may influence a whole cascade of regulatory activities.

1.2 Proliferative Phase

The second phase of wound repair is characterized by proliferation, therefore called the proliferative or regenerative phase. This lasts from day 1 after wounding to a maximum of 14 days.

Granulation Tissue Formation

Highly vascularized tissue is formed; in addition to leukocytes which are the dominant cells in the inflammatory phase, histiocytes, fibrocytes, fibroblasts, plasma cells, mast cells, angioblasts, and myofibroblasts move into the site of the lesion.

Wound Edema, a Starting Signal for Fibroblasts

As a consequence of activated leukocytes adhering to endothelial cells and bradykinin release from mast cells, vascular permeability increases, substances of large molecular weight (albumin, fibrinogen) diffuse into the extracellular space, leading to edema.

Fluid accumulation is a specific trigger transforming fibrocytes into fibroblasts, inducing cell proliferation, and therefore leading to rapid granulation tissue formation. This dynamic tissue change is fundamental for epithelialization. It consists of capillary sprouts, newly built capillaries, and fibroblasts. Fibroblasts migrate and proliferate during the whole healing process using amino acids, derived from lysed blood clots in the wound, as substrates.

Angiogenesis

It is known today that cells from the venous endothelium are the first to respond to angiogenic stimuli and start to migrate.

Cytoplasmic pseudopods move between fragmented basal membranes. Endothelial cells follow. Their loss is compensated by proliferation of endothelial cells within the vessel of origin. Another track for endothelial migration is fibronectin synthezised by blood vessels.

Myofibroblasts

Myofibroblasts are modified fibroblasts which closely resemble smooth muscle cells in structure. They contain contractile fibers. Granulation tissue contains indeed as much actinomyosin as the uterus of a pregnant rat.

The wound surface is reduced by myofibroblast contraction. Presumably the cells communicate via cell-to-cell contact or substrate.

Collagen fibril maturation contributes very little to wound contraction. Due to contraction, wound margins are approximated 1–2 mm per day. However, wound contraction does not play as decisive a role in the healing process in humans as it does in animals.

Fibronectin

Fibronectin is essential to the outcome of the proliferative phase. This glycoprotein is found on cell surfaces, on connective tissue matrix, and in extracellular fluid. It causes adhesion of cells to the fibrin matrix but also has chemotactic capacities, which regulates cell movement.

1.3 Reparative Phase

During the last phase of wound healing the production of new connective tissue is of main importance. As soon as fibroblasts synthesize collagen fibrils, their mitotic activity is turned off. Cell density and vascularization of the wound decrease, while collagen fibrils mature. Scar formation is initiated. Both collagen deposition and fibroblast orientation is determined by fibronectin, which constitutes most of the extracellular matrix at this stage of repair.

Hyaluronic Acid Enhances Cell Motility and Mitosis

Cell movement in newly formed granulation tissue depends on the presence of hyaluronic acid:

11

– It facilitates adhesion and separation of contacts between cell laminae and ground substance.

– It leads to swelling by massive hydratation creating space between collagen fibrils and cells

Proteoglycans

These molecules consist of one core protein covalently bound to at least one glucosaminoglycan (mucopolysaccharide). Chondroitin-4-sulfate improves polymerization of collagen monomers in vitro. Heparan sulfate binds cell substrate within the wound. As with hyaluronic acid and collagen, proteoglycans are continuously being resynthesized during wound repair.

Collagen

In a healing wound collagen type III predominates. Collagen type V increases analogously to neovascularization. There is a strong correlation between endothelial cells and type V collagen. Wound disruption strength is still poor: 3 weeks after wounding the fresh scar has approximately 20 % of final strength. The increase overtime is achieved not only by collagen accumulation but also by the restructuring of collagen.

Epithelialization

If all epidermal layers are affected, epithelialization is initiated from the wound margins. In superficial wounds, where the basal cell layer is intact, the damaged area can be reconstructed by mitosis of remaining cells, differentiating into mature epidermis.

Stages of Epithelialization

Reepithelialization proceeds through the following three stages: migration of basal lamina cells, mitosis of cells migrating across the wound surface, and maturation of newly generated cells.

Migration of Epithelial Cells

Early after tissue injury desmosomes, which provide mechanical stability of the epithelial unit in healthy skin, detach. In their cytoplasma keratinocytes produce peripheral actin fibrils. Additional tonofibril retraction makes possible cell movement. About 24 h after wounding cells from the basal cell layer move in an amoeboid manner across the wound area. They migrate on top of the basal lamina or, in the case of disruption, on a temporary lamina consisting of fibronectin, type V collagen, and fibrin.

Keratinocytes Construct Their Own Matrix

Besides the capacity to move, keratinocytes are able to synthesize fibronectin. As mentioned above, fibronectin forms a provisional matrix along which cells migrate. Already during cell migration this temporary basal lamina is transformed into its final form by producing type IV collagen and laminin.

Migratory Stimuli for Epithelial Cells

In epithelial damage cells loose contact. This initiates migration. Consequently, migration stops as soon as cells regain contact on all sides during wound closure (Fig. 7). The new basal lamina is constructed step by step: the first cell remains on the surface of the wound (so-called "self implantation"), the second moves on top and stays there, followed by the next which sits on top of the second one etc. ("leap-frog hypothesis").

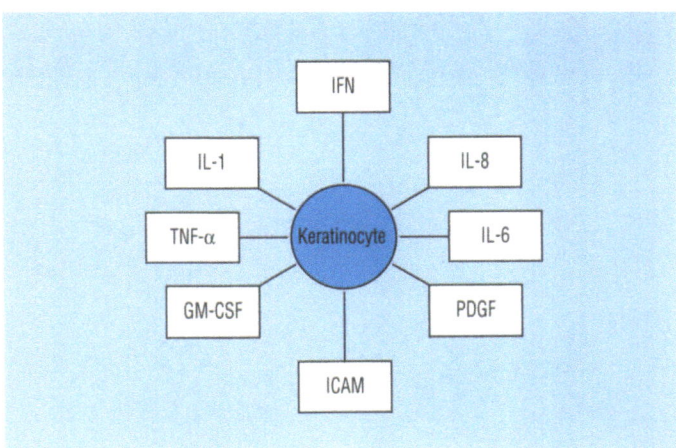

Fig. 6.
Cytokines and growth factors secreted by keratinocytes

Fig. 7. Epithelial
migration

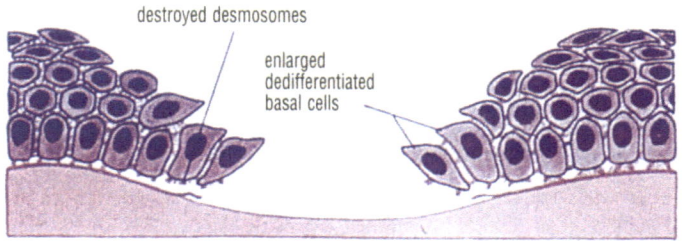

destroyed desmosomes

enlarged
dedifferentiated
basal cells

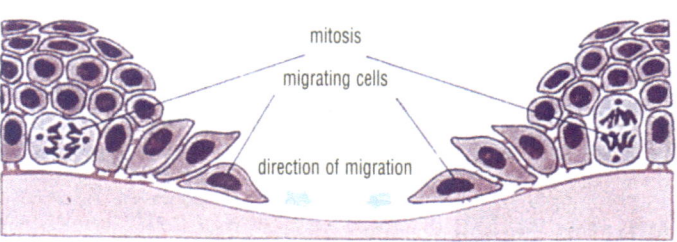

mitosis

migrating cells

direction of migration

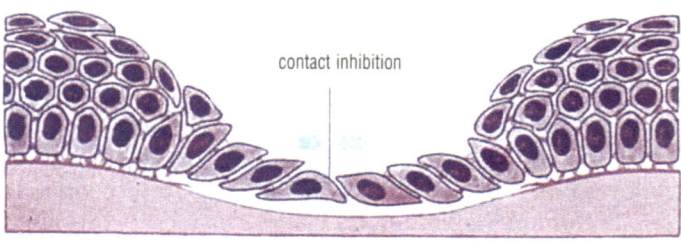

contact inhibition

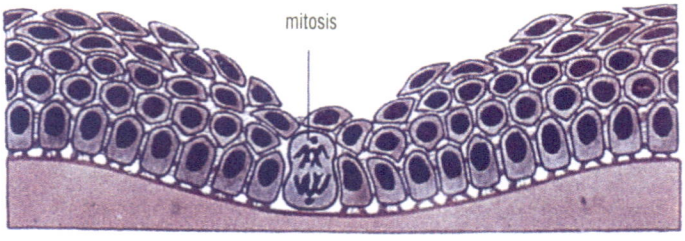

mitosis

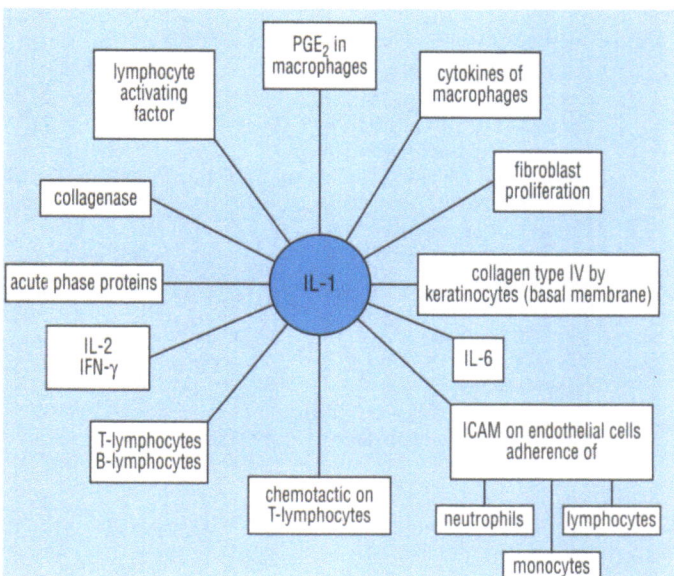

Fig. 8.
Effects of IL-1 in
wound healing

Only basal lamina cells are capable of DNA production and of cell division. Cell migration and proliferation are processes occurring at the same time but independently of one another.

Basal Cells Divide

Mitotic activity of basal cells close to the damage site increases 12–48 h after wounding. Mature epidermis usually produces chalones inhibiting mitosis, which regulate cell proliferation. In a wound the epidermis function is impaired and therefore synthesizes no chalones. The missing inhibitory effect of mitosis stimulates remaining cells to proliferate (negative feedback mechanism).

Stimulation of Mitosis

Various factors, such as EGF and FGF stimulate mitosis, therefore influencing both epithelialization and granulation.

Interleukins

IL-1 has a stimulatory effect on mitosis. IL-1 triggers T-lymphocytes to produce IL-2, which activates T- and B-lymphocytes, granulocytes, monocytes, and natural killer cells and stimulates fibroblast proliferation (Fig. 8).

Activities of keratinocytes during wound healing

1. Formation of new epidermis
   a. Phenotypic changes
   - retraction of tonofibrils
   - detachment of desmosomes
   - shaping of peripheral cytoplasmic actin fibrils
   b. Migration across wound surface
   c. Growth of regular epidermis
   - stratum corneum functions as permeability barrier
   - tonofibrils and desmosomes (disruption strength)
   - basal lamina (firm junction to dermis)
2. Secretion of biologically active substances
   a. Vasoactive mediators
   b. Growth factors
   c. Proteases and other enzymes
   d. Macromolecules forming epithelial structure

1.4 Epithelial Maturation

The final step in epidermal wound healing is characterized by cell maturation – leading to regeneration of a defined epidermal layer. During these cell differentiation processes enzymatic metabolism is markedly enhanced. The key enzyme is ornithine decarboxylase.

The glycogen, RNA, and DNA content of epithelial cells increases. Keratinization starts, and finally desmosomes promote attachment of cells to one another. The wound is closed and covered by mature epidermis.

2 Impaired Wound Healing

Deficiently healing wounds are characterized by missing or insufficient, retarded wound closure.

Characteristics of deficient wound healing

Retarded wound closure
Detritus
Pus
Insufficient arterial circulation
Reduced venous return
Vasculitis, vasculitis of capillary network
Wound infection

2.1 Local Factors Contributing to Impaired Wound Healing

Wound infection is indicated by detritus (scab, necrotic material, fibrin aggregates) and pus. Frequently observed vascular components are reduced venous return, insufficient arterial circulation, vasculitis in general or vasculitis of the capillary network. Furthermore, the wound may be contaminated with bacteria, fungi, or viruses. All cited conditions can lead finally to metabolic impairment thus delaying wound closure.

2.2 Systemic Conditions Affecting Wound Repair

2.2.1 Protein Deficiency

Regenerating tissue requires amino acids for protein synthesis and as an energy source for gluconeogenesis. Thus, the consequences of protein deficiency are:
- Reduced humoral and cell-mediated immunity
- Impaired phagocytosis and bacterial killing
- Reduced collagen synthesis

In hypoalbuminemic edema the distance of nutrient diffusion is increased.

2.2.2 Vitamin Deficiency

Vitamin A

Vitamin A is essential for glycoprotein and proteoglycan synthesis. Vitamin A deficiency leads to:

- Retarded epithelialization
- Retarded collagen synthesis
- Reduced collagen stability
- Recurrent, serious infections

Vitamin C

Collagen synthesis requires vitamin C for hydroxylation of proline and lysine. As capillary integrity depends on formation of stable collagen types III and IV, vitamin C deficiency leads to capillary fragility. Further consequences of vitamin C deficiency are:

- Impaired macrophage migration
- Decreased neutrophil function
- Reduced complement and immunoglobulin synthesis

Because humans cannot store vitamin C, chronically ill patients are likely to acquire vitamin C deficiency.

Vitamin K

Vitamin K deficiency can affect wound regeneration through vitamin K dependent coagulation factors. If there is a shortage in prothrombin or factor VII, IX, or X, bleeding and bacterial superinfection of the wound area may occur.

Vitamin B

Vitamin B deficiency may impair wound healing only in animals. Wounds show less disruption strength than those of normal animals.

Vitamin E

The role of vitamin E in burn wounds has not yeet been defined.

2.2.3 Hyperbilirubinemia

In vitro and in animal models hyperbilirubinemia prohibits wound healing by reducing fibroblast proliferation.

2.2.4 Factor XIII

Fibrin-consuming diseases such as colitis ulcerosa, burns, rheumatoid arthritis, acute leukemia, and Crohn's disease are accompanied by reduced factor XIII activity. Factor XIII also seems to be involved in certain vascular diseases such as chronic venous insufficiency; in Klippel-Trenaunay syndrome factor XIII deficiency is acquired.

The clinical relevance of this phenomenon remains to be clarified. Factor XIII binds fibronectin to collagen and transforms urea-soluble fibrin into its unsoluble form. For this reason it plays a role in wound healing. Factor XIII substitution enhances wound repair and fracture healing. Individuals with congenital factor XIII deficiency show delayed wound regeneration. In contrast, some authors report inhibitory effects of factor XIII on epithelialization.

2.2.5 Drugs Affecting Wound Repair

The following medications may act considerably on healing:

Glucocorticoids. Inhibit: granulation tissue formation, epidermal regeneration, macrophage chemotaxis, fibroblast proliferation, prostaglandin synthesis, glycosaminoglycan synthesis. Stimulate: Collagen degradation, neovascularization.

Cytostatics. Especially alkylating cytostatics are regarded as inhibitors of wound healing.

Cyclosporin. Theoretically, one might expect cyclosporin to have a similar, negative effect on wound healing as glucocorticoids. Preliminary studies on wound disruption strength under cyclosporin treatment confirm this.

Colchicine. Colchicine leads to vasoconstriction, therefore reducing circulation in the wound area; it inhibits collagen synthesis and consequently reduces the collagen content in the wound.

Penicillinamine. Collagen stability and wound disruption strength are diminuished due to inhibition of the metallo-enzyme lysyl-oxidase, which cross-links collagen.

Calcitonin. In a rabbit animal model intramuscular calcitonine application enhances protein synthesis, keratinocyte proliferation, and collagen production.

2.2.6 Further Wound Healing Risk Factors

Age

Age has an influence on all phases of wound repair:
- Wound contraction is reduced
- Cell proliferation is diminished
- Neovascularization is reduced
- Number of mast cells is decreased
- Epithelialization is slowed
- Keratinocytes proliferate to a lesser extent following mitogenic stimuli

Rare Connective Tissue Diseases

Ehlers-Danlos syndrome and proline hydroxylase deficiency lead to wound healing impairment.

3 Chronic Wounds

Which wounds fall under the category unsatisfactory healing? Examples include leg ulcers, decubitus, pyoderma gangrenosum, ecthymata, superinfected, surgical wounds, chemical burns, and burn wounds.

Definition

A poorly healing wound is defined as any kind of wound which does not heal within the biological time range of 2–3 weeks. The only exceptions are large open wounds healing from the wound margin; under normal conditions it takes longer for these wounds to completely re epithelialize.

3.1 Pressure Sores

A continuous change in weight distribution during standing, sitting, and lying achieved by movement must be regarded as a physiological protective mechanism. This permits healthy persons to prevent long-lasting, inadequate pressure on certain exposed parts of their body. If the mechanism is impaired such as in diseases of the central nervous system, the peripheral nervous system (lesions of the spinal cord, cerebral insult), posttrauma, and in the elderly, the permanent pressure on skin and underlying tissues leads to necrosis and to a pressure sore (decubitus ulcer).

3.1.1 Pathogenesis

The cause of pressure sores was not recognized for a long time although it is a very simple concept. Continuous pressure on one specific area is the main pathophysiological mechanism. The more intense the pressure the earlier a lesion emerges, which means there is an inverse relationship between pressure intensity and application time. If tissue compression is below a capillary pressure of 45 mmHg, small venules become occluded. The region of impaired circulation becomes clinically apparent as an erythema; this process is reversible.

If the applied pressure is higher than a capillary pressure of 45 mmHg, arterioles close and the area becomes ischemic. Depending on time (e.g., 70 mmHg for 2 h), tissue damage is irreversible. In the beginning, necrosis is found in subcutis and underlying muscle; later the skin becomes affected. Studies have shown that necrotic areas are a preferable site of bacterial infection. Manifest infection is a common complication in ulcer disease.

Incidence and Risk Factors

Pressure sores occur in certain exposed areas: sacrum, ischium, greater trochanter, fibular head, lateral and medial malleolus, and heel. More than 80% of all pressure sores and ulcers are found at these sites. In individuals whose sensibility and/or mobility is reversibly reduced such as in intoxicated, traumatized, or anesthesized patients or irreversibly destroyed such as in para- or tetraplegic patients, the risk of pressure sores is even greater. The incidence of decubitus in this patient group is 44% to 86%, which is ten times greater than in the overall population. The elderly also present a significant susceptibility to pressure sores: 71% of pressure sore patients are older than 70 years, and 8.8% of those living in an old people's homes suffer from chronic ulcer. The reasons for this include catabolic metabolism, immobility, and incontinence. Some 3%–4% of all hospitalized patients develop pressure sores. As a result the complication and mortality rate is 8%. Various scales have been developed to calculate the risk of pressure sore formation in hospitalized patients. One of these is the Norton scale, based on mental condition, activity, and mobility (Table 1); these evaluation criteria are graded by points. Using the Norton scale, it has been shown that patients with a low risk (18–20 points) move 110–225 times while sleeping, whereas high-risk patients (14 or fewer points) change position only 2–20 times during the same period of time. Based on the Norton scale prophylactic treatment can be initiated early.

Table 1. Clinical scoring system (Norton scale: risk for developing a pressure sore at 14 points or below)

General physical condition		Mental state		Activity		Mobility		Inconti- nence	
Good	4	Alert	4	Ambulant	4	Full	4	Normal function	4
Fair	3	Apathetic	3	Walks with help	3	Slightly limited	3	Occa- sionally	3
Poor	2	Confused	2	Chair- bound	2	Very limited	2	Usually (urine)	2
Bad	1	Stuporous	1	Bedbound	1	Im- mobile	1	Urine and feces	1

(Maximum score = 20)

Clinical Stages of Pressure Sores

Four stages are distinguished:

Stage I: Erythema, reversible hyperemia

Stage II: Superficial; aching, blistering accompanied by blue, livid color of skin, reaches epidermis and dermis

Stage III: Deep ulcer, edema and inflammation of margin, reaches bony process

Stage IV: Extensive ulcus; involvement of bone, bursae, joint or cavities (e.g., rectum, vagina; Fig. 9)

In addition, noninfected ulcers must be differentiated from infected ones. Adequate conservative and/or surgical thera- peutic concepts are indicated according to the ulcer stage.

Fig. 9.
Decubitus, stage IV

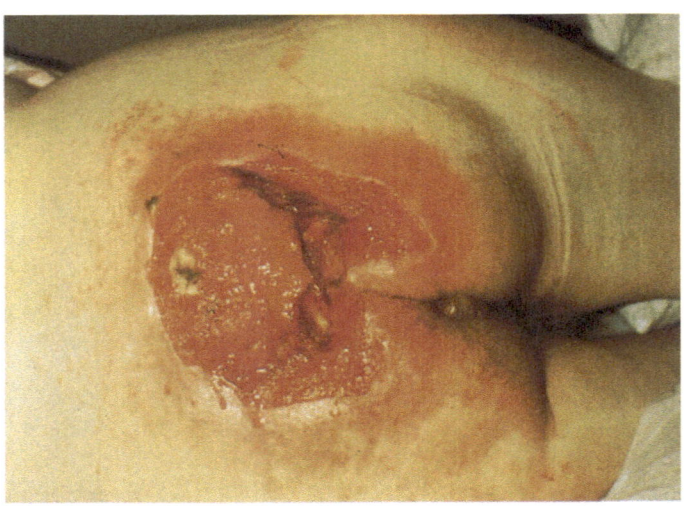

Pressure Sore Prevention

The major concern in dealing with patients who are likely to develop pressure sores must be prevention. Three basic principles must be regarded:

- Long-lasting pressure on predisposed areas must be prevented.
- Measures to enhance tissue perfusion should be applied.
- Risk factors must be reduced; primary disease must be treated.

To be evaluate the risk of the individual patient, clinical scores such as the Norton scale (see above) should be used. It is important repeatedly to check certain parameters of the patient (at least once or twice per week), to recognize changes in the patient's state and possibly to adapt treatment.

Positioning of the patient: The most effective prevention is mobilizing the patient. If this is impossible, the patient's position should be changed at regular time intervals by the nursing staff; to decrease the duration a certain force is exerted. The following sequence is well established: Supine position – 30° right lateral position – supine position – 30° left lateral position – supine position. The time interval should be 2 h. If breathing is not affected, the patient may also be turned into a prone position.

Pressure dispersion devices: The main objective is to disperse pressure over a greater surface area thus extending the length of time that the force may be applied. The patient should be placed on a particularly soft bed. This includes heel and ankle protection using heel caps or boots or by positioning the lower extremities in such a way that they do not touch the bed. Air pillow cushions, sheep skin, and foam material minimize shear and pressure to these areas. In high-risk patients special pressure-dispersing beds have proven successful. Systems such as the laminar flow bed and air pillow cushion beds (Table 2) allow pressure reduction below the capillary perfusion level (<45 mmHg).

Table 2. Pressure on the skin surface using different methods of pressure dispersion (recordings in mmHg; adapted from Chicarilli)

Air-fluidized bed	30 (mean 18–25)
Low-air-loss bed	32 (mean 18–25)
Feather pillows on foam	36
Water bed	58
Foam mattress	68
Spring mattress	164
Operating table	140–260

Enhancement of Tissue Perfusion

Improving peripheral circulation is an additional, very important goal which should be included in systematic pressure prevention. This is achieved by active and passive physiotherapy, mobilization of the patient by sitting, and if possible walking with assistance. Training equipment such as an expander to exercise upper arm and shoulder muscles when the lower half of the body is parallized must be available. Roborants and periodic refreshening of the skin are indicated. This includes gently rubbing predisposed areas with crushed ice, then drying them with a soft towel or a hair dryer. Daily skin care and cleaning procedures, especially in incontinent patients, are also part of prophylaxis. Moisturizing lotions at neutral pH and skin protection creams avoid dry skin. Bed linen must be clean and without folds.

Treatment of Risk Factors and Primary Disease

Treatment of the primary disease, deficiencies (e.g., vitamins) and metabolic diseases is of main importance. Enteral nutrition must be maintained as long as possible; if active oral food uptake is insufficient, duodenal tube feeding should be maintained until parenteral feeding is unavoidable. Various experimental and clinical studies have shown that enteral nutrition is superior to parenteral. The latter must be used as for only as short a time as possible, substituting calories according to the daily nutritional requirements as well as minerals and vitamins.

3.1.2 Therapy

Once a pressure sore develops, there are both conservative and aggressive ways to treat it. The decision regarding how to treat depends on the clinical stage of the necrosis and the primary disease of the patient. If immobilization is only temporary, such as after a heart attack or trauma, conservative treatment is indicated. In these patients surgical intervention should be performed at the earliest after 6 months if the ulcer does not heal. In contrast, a parallized patient, for example, one with a spinal cord lesion showing a deeply penetrating large decubitus ulcer, would be considered a candidate for surgical closure.

Conservative Management

Conservative therapy is determined with regard to the severity of the ulcer and is based on five principles (adapted from Seiler):

– Pressure relief
– Removal of necrotic material (débridement)
– Infection control
– Wound dressing
– Minimizing risk factors

The most crucial first step is removing off the pressure from irritated areas of the body. In decubitus ulcer stage I, the wound shows restitutio ad integrum within 1 h. In consequence, the interval of positioning change is shortened, the skin is kept clean and dry, and the sheets are checked to remain smooth and uncreased.

A stage II pressure sore should have a minimum of 36 h of pressure relief by frequently changing the patient's position. A particulary soft underlying surface must be chosen. Infection control is important; bacterial culture should be performed regularly. Colorless antiseptics (e.g., hydrogen peroxide) should be preferred. The wound dressing must provide a moist environment such as semipermeable dressings do. If there is consistent pressure relief, stage II lesions should be reversible. In long-term immobilized patients, a more sophisticated pressure-dispersing system should be employed in the form of an air-fluidized or low-air-loss bed.

Conservative treatment of the extensive stage III decubitus ulcer always involves accurate surgical débridement, which is performed with a surgical spoon and scalpel. If nonviable tissue is not removed from the wound, it can serve as a medium for bacterial proliferation. The simple wound contamination must be distinguished from wound infection. In general, all decubiti demonstrate a variety of microbial flora. Germ concentrations greater than 10^5 per gram tissue lead to manifest infections and impaired wound healing. There is a strong association between germ concentrations in excess of 10^9 per gram tissue and systemic sepsis. Gram-negative bacteria such as *Proteus mirabilis* and *Pseudomonas aeruginosa*, anaerobes such as Bacteroids and gram-positives such as *Staphylococcus aureus* are frequently found. Mixed infections are common. In the case of systemic infection the choice of antibiotics should be based on proven antibacterial efficiency.

Just as important as surgical débridement is the defined application of certain local therapeutics and dressings. Proteolytic enzymes (Table 3) may be used to support débridement and cleansing of the wound. As some of these are available in combination with antibiotics, sensitization and resistance must be taken into consideration when used

Table 3. Proteolytic enzymes in wound healing

Enzyme	Antibiotic
Trypsin	+ Framycetin sulfate
Plasmin + deoxyribonuclease	
Streptokinase + streptodornase	
Collagenase	+ Chloramphenicol

Fig. 10a–c.
Decubitus ulcer.
a Before therapy.
b Seven days after
therapy.
c Twenty-one days
after therapy with
1.2 U collagenase

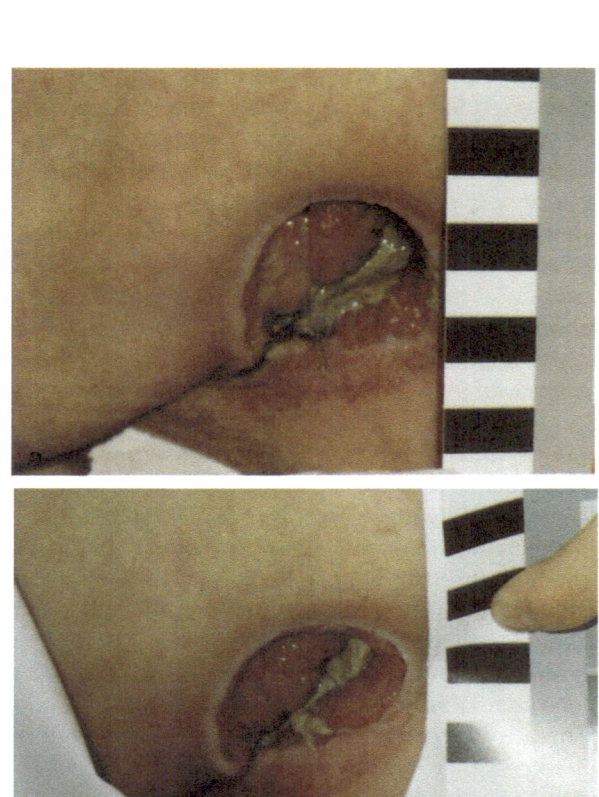

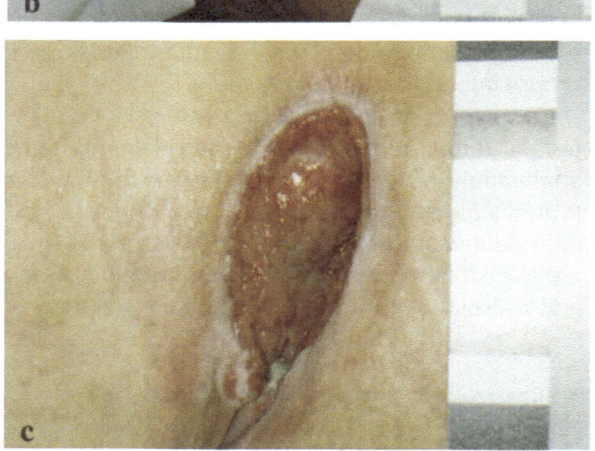

frequently. Collagenase has the advantage of specifically cleaving human collagen. Cleavage products act chemotactically on macrophages and fibroblasts thus promoting granulation tissue formation (Fig. 10).

Following surgical and enzymatic débridement, the clean wound is conditioned, which means granulation tissue formation is enhanced. Moist semiocclusive dressings are generally the most beneficial. To effect osmosis, either sugar or hypertonic sodium chloride (20 %) pads may be placed on the wound. A recently developed treatment strategy is to activate macrophages by covering the wound with compresses soaked with tetrachlorodecaoxide (TCDO, diluted 1 : 5 with 0.9 % sodium chloride). Optimal occlusive conditions are achieved by using semipermeable membranes (e.g. hydrocolloids). Depending on ulcer size, wound dressings may be required for months. Small ulcers should heal spontaneuosly if systematic pressure relief is ensured. Wound closure can be accelerated by split skin grafting (mesh graft), which can be performed in regional anesthesia in small lesions.

Surgical Therapy

Usually wound closure in stage III and IV pressure sores can be obtained only by surgery. The first measure is to excise the ulcer completely and, if necessary, to perform partial ostectomy (ischium, greater trochanter) or/and bursectomy (sacrum, greater trochanter). Primary wound closure should always be preferred by mobilizing healthy tissue and direct suturing of the wound margins. In non paraplegic patients the ulcer is prepared for a mesh graft. If this is not successful, flap plasties are a suitable alternative. The workhorse of surgical management of pressure sores is the random skin flap: the flap is elevated in a plane between subcutaneous tissue and deep fascia, then advanced or rotated into the defect. In sacral pressure sores the ulcer cavity is covered with a bilateral buttock rotation flap (Fig. 11). A complication rate of 15 % including hematoma, flap necrosis, and infection has been reported in the literature. During the past decade myocutaneous flaps have been established as an alternative. These flaps are elevated in a plane beneath the muscle-saving musculocutaneous perforators to the overlying skin. These may also be transferred as free flaps if they possess an adequate vascular pedicle, to be reanastomosed using microvascular techniques. The advantages of musculocutaneous flaps are: a higher blood flow

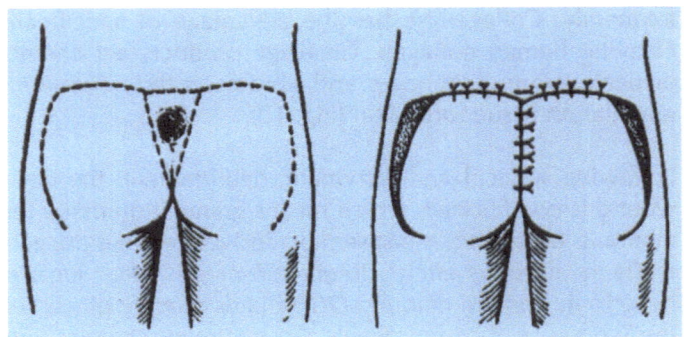

rate provides enhanced resistance to bacterial invasion, and large defects can be closed due to the increased flap bulk. In paraplegic patients with nonhealing sacral pressure sores the intercostal or sensory island flap is an attractive solution since it allows sensory transfer to a previously anesthetic area. The flap is elevated over the T9–10 interspace with extreme care of preserving the lateral cutanous nerve branch and tunneled to the sacral defect. The restoration of sensibility in this area helps to prevent recurrent pressure sore development. In paraplegics the relapse rate is less than with other flap techniques.

Trochanteric pressure sores can be approached surgically with lateral thigh rotation flaps or the very reliable myocutaneous tensor fascia lata flap. Bursectomy and osteotomy of bony prominences (trochanter) are necessary components of deleting localized pressure projection. In severe cases with pyarthrosis of the hip joint (stage IV) amputation is the adequate surgical therapy. A reasonable alternative may be improvement of the patient's general condition and acceptance of the pyarthrosis as a permanent situation.

In advanced ischial ulcers the bursal sac is part of the ulcus cavity. The ischial tuberosity is likely to become a source of chronic ostitis. The most reliable random flap is the posterior thigh flap, which is rotated cranially into the crater. The biceps femoris muscle is commonly used as padding after partial ostectomy of the ischium. For this the biceps may be divided inferiorly. Vascular integrity is maintained by preserving most of the superior perforating veins.

Due to poor long-term results – especially paraplegics show recurrences in the form of perineal and scrotal pressure sores – total ischiectomy is very rarely performed. If complications occur, they are very difficult to treat in a secondary surgical approach. Therefore it is recommended to perform partial ostectomy removing diseased bone and flattening the offending pressure point.

An alternative flap in the ischial region is the tensor fascia lata myocutaneous flap.

3.2 Chronic Leg Ulcer

3.2.1 Differential Diagnosis

Causes of leg ulceration

Venous
Arterial
Chronic peripheral arterial occlusive disease
Arteriolar ulcers
Necrotic angiodermitis
Hypertensive (Martorell's) ulcer
Diabetic microulcers
(Necrobiosis lipoidica, "pretibial pigmented patches")
Embolic ulcers
Vasculitic ulcers
Superficial vasculitis
Livedo vasculitis
Pyoderma gangrenosum
Periarteritis nodosa
Wegener's granulomatosis

Chronic Leg Ulcer Is a Symptom

Chronic leg ulcer (crural ulcer) should not be regarded as a diagnosis but a polyetiological symptom. Although 85% of leg ulcers are venous in origin, other possible causes should always be taken into consideration.

Chronic Peripheral Arterial Occlusive Disease

The most common cause of nonvenous leg ulcers is chronic peripheral arterial occlusive disease, including endarteritis obliterans and arteriosclerosis obliterans. Arterial ulcers are localized mainly in areas of the lower leg which are exposed to trivial injuries. Recent studies indicate that tissue damage may be a result of toxic mediators released by leukocytes which are activated by ischemia and increased adherence to capillary endothelium.

Small Vessel Disease

In some cases periarteritis nodosa is cause of an arterial leg ulcer. Small arteries and arterioles are damaged in diabetic microangiopathy and necrobiosis lipoidica diabeticorum.

The latter is characterized histologically by fibrinoid insudation and arterial swelling. Typical localization is the ventral aspect of the lower leg.

Hypertensive Martorell's Ulcer

The cause of hypertensive (Martorell's) ulcer is subendo-thelial hyaline degeneration of small arteries. As a consequence of hypertension, which is essential for diagnosis, the thickness of intima and media increases, and the vessel diameter is reduced. This ulcer type is located at the ventral or lateral aspect of the lower leg. Often they are found symmetrically on opposite sides.

Aneurysm

Very rarely ulcers result from arterial aneurysms with dislodged thrombotic material, embolizing peripheral arteries in the lower leg.

Ulcers in Vasculitis

Patients with vasculitis usually show small ulcers on both lower legs (about the size of a coin). Depending on the localization of vasculitis, ulcers are superficial (superficial vasculitis) or deep (deep vasculitis). Pyoderma gangrenosum is a specific type of vasculitic ulcer characterized by a muddy, necrotic wound surface with undermined margins and extreme painfulness.

Exogenous Leg Ulcers

Exogenous crural ulcers are caused by physical or chemical trauma. They must be differentiated from ulcers of infectious origin. Infectious ulcers were earlier seen in lupus vulgaris, lues stage III, and leprosy. Nowadays in developed countries the most common infectious ulcers are staphylococcus-associated ecthyma with "punched-out" undermined wound margins. Additionally, erysipelas may necrotise and cause leg ulcer formation.

Hematological Diseases

Hematological diseases such as sickle cell anemia, spherocytic anemia, thalassemia, glucose-6-phosphate dehydrogenase deficiency, factor XIII deficiency, and essential thrombocytosis may contribute to the development of a leg ulcer. It is not known whether thrombophilia caused by a hematological disease may lead to phlebothrombosis with consequent development of chronic venous insufficiency and chronic leg ulcer.

Chronic ulcers which do not heal in spite of sufficient long-term treatment are always suspicious of being neoplastic in nature. Such lesions are seen in ulcerating basiloma, spinocellular carcinoma, soft-tissue sarcoma, hemangio-endothelioma, malignant lymphoma and malignant melanoma. Benign neoplasms such as hemangioma, pre-cancerous lesions, and hisiocytoma may ulcerate and create chronic leg ulcers.

Marjolin's Ulcer

Long-term chronic inflammation such as osteomyelitis or skin damage due to irradiation (radiodermatitis) may lead to degeneration and malignant ulcer transformation. Such a lesion is called Marjolin's ulcer.

The great variety of possible causes proves that a chronic leg ulcer is only a symptom. Establishing the correct diagnosis is therefore always a great challenge for every physician.

3.2.2 Chronic Venous Insufficiency

Chronic venous insufficiency may be epifascial or sub-fascial. This depends on the exact site of valve damage, either above or beneath the muscular fascia.

Subfascial Venous Insufficiency

The most common cause of subfascial venous insufficiency is deep vein thrombosis. Although 80% of thrombotic occlusions are recanalized within 1 year, total restitution of the damaged valves is rarely achieved. In most cases correct valve function is irreversibly lost. Venous return is diminished. The direction of blood is reversed, which is called pendulum flow. As a consequence there is a volume-dependent increase in pressure load in the deep venous system. This causes insufficiency of the vein valves of the perforating veins. Blood flowing from subfascial to epifascial veins may lead to development of secondary epifascial varicosis.

Localization of Thrombosis Determines Subsequent Damage

The degree to which chronic venous insufficiency produces subsequent damage is determined mainly by the site of thrombosis. Patients with iliac venous thrombosis develop leg edema, but never leg ulcers as long as distal veins remain competent. In contrast, thrombosis of the popliteal vein or the paired veins of the lower leg may cause early signs of chronic venous insufficiency.

Insufficiency of Subfascial Veins Is a Common Disease

Subfascial venous insufficiency may occur secondary to thrombosis, but also as a primary disease in association with hereditary valve agenesis, valve hypoplasia, or primary degeneration of subfascial veins leading to varicosis. The hemodynamic and clinical consequences are identical with those seen in postthrombotic subfascial venous insufficiency.

Epifascial Venous Insufficiency

Epifascial venous insufficiency presents clinically as superficial varicosis. It is important to differentiate between insufficiency of the main saphenous veins (great and small saphenous vein), isolated insufficiency of venous branches, and reticular varicosis. Insufficient saphenous veins communicate with the subfascial veins via perforating veins and venae communicantes. However, isolated insufficiency of venous branches may exist without insufficiency of perforating veins.

Complete Varicosis of the Great Saphenous Vein

Varicosis of the great saphenous vein may be classified as complete and incomplete varicosis. By definition complete varicosis is diagnosed when the proximal site of insufficiency occurs at the groin. Depending on the length of the insufficient vessel, varicosis is divided into stage I (reflux 10 cm distal from the groin), stage II (reflux down to the proximal knee), stage III (reflux down to the lower leg), and stage IV (reflux down to the medial malleolus).

In incomplete varicosis of the great saphenous vein no reflux is detectable in the groin area. Instead, an insufficient perforating vein causes increasing reflux via the great saphenous vein to distal veins. This most common type of incomplete varicosis is called the perforating type of incomplete varicosis of the great saphenous vein.

Fig. 12.
Stages of varicosis
of the great
saphenous vein

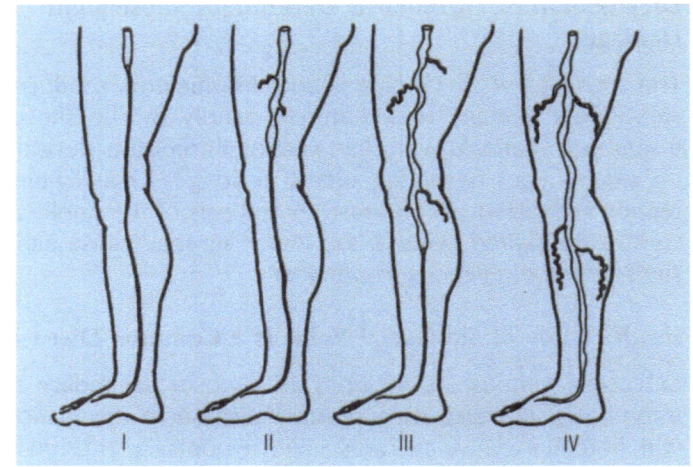

Small Saphenous Vein

Varicosis of the small saphenous vein is divided in the same manner: in complete varicosis of the small saphenous vein reflux is present at the conjunction between the small saphenous vein and the popliteal vein. Stage I is defined by reflux up to 10 cm distally, stage II by reflux down to the distal lower leg, and stage III by reflux down to the lateral malleolus.

Incomplete varicosis of the smaller saphenous vein is characterized by reflux distal to the popliteal area, where valves are still intact.

Clinical Prognosis of Insufficiency of the Different Venous Systems

The prognosis of of chronic valvular insufficiency differs according to its location. The best prognosis is in isolated lateral vein varicosis and reticular varicosis since communication to subfascial veins is not lacking. Complications are seen very rarely.

Valvular insufficiency of the saphenous veins and of perforating veins may lead to typical signs of chronic venous insufficiency. In healthy individuals about 10% of the venous return from the lower extremities flows through epifascial veins. Depending on the severity of impairment in isolated varicosis of the saphenous veins, excess blood volume may escape through intact perforating veins into the subfascial venous system.

Severe complications of chronic venous insufficieny such as venous leg ulcer are not seen in varicosis of saphenous veins, as long as there is no additional incompetence of perforating veins.

If perforating veins are insufficient, orthograde venous return is irreversibly damaged. As a consequence of subsequent venous hypertension and volume overload epifascial veins become dilated and valves lose their function. The prognosis is worse. Venous ulcers are found typically in the area of Cockett's veins, which are located proximal to the medial malleolus.

Cockett's perforating veins are likely to become insufficient. There are three known reasons:

- They are located very distally and therefore are subject to maximum hemodynamic pressure.

- They are relatively short, direct connections between superficial and deep veins without intermediate muscles in between. More proximal perforating veins join the deep venous system mostly via muscle veins, passing the fascia diagonally. With each muscle contraction the fascia is dislocated, obstructing perforating veins. This does not happen in Cockett's veins.

- Cockett's veins often join a lateral posterior vein with a fragile venous wall more susceptible to dilatation, instead of the greater saphenous vein, which could compensate retrograde pressure to some extent.

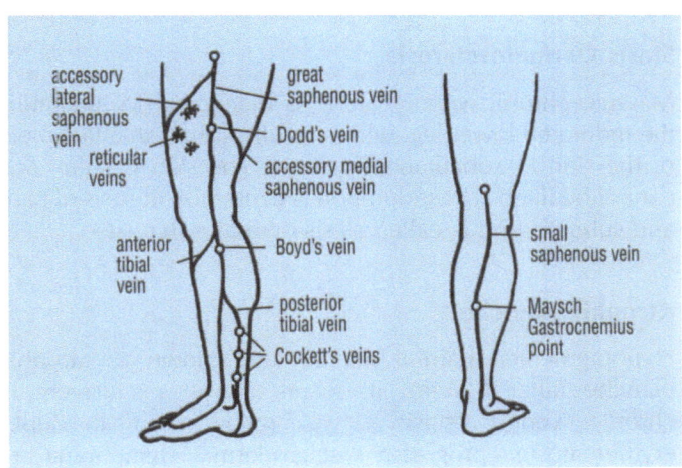

accessory lateral saphenous vein
reticular veins
great saphenous vein
Dodd's vein
accessory medial saphenous vein
anterior tibial vein
Boyd's vein
posterior tibial vein
Cockett's veins
small saphenous vein
Maysch Gastrocnemius point

Fig. 13. Anatomy of superficial leg veins and Cockett's perforating veins

Insufficiency of Deep Veins

Insufficiency of the deep venous system has the worst prognosis. Under physiological conditions 90% of the venous blood from the lower extremities runs through the deep venous system. Therefore insufficiency results in an immense volume overload, leading to insufficiency of perforating veins and varicosis of epifascial veins. The hemodynamics is severely disturbed. In this condition the postthrombotic syndrom is the most common cause of leg ulcer.

3.2.3 Clinical Features and Pathogenesis of Ulcus Cruris Venosum

The skin is the main target organ damaged by chronic venous insufficiency. By definition, there are three stages of chronic venous stasis.

Chronic Venous Insufficiency Stage I

Typical signs of stage I venous stasis are enlargement of cutaneous veins (especially at the ankle and lateral sole of the foot), erythema, and ankle edema. During phlebological examination the patient must also be inspected from behind to recognize discrete signs of beginning edema.

Chronic Venous Insufficiency Stage II (Fig. 14)

With advancing venous stasis edema increases around the tibia. Brown to yellow pigmented macula are found on the lower leg, called purpura jaune d'ocre or dermite ocre.

Stasis Dermatosclerosis

Massive chronic venous stasis is diagnosed by palpating the indurated lower leg, which results from firm attachment of the skin to subcutaneous tissue. The skin is shiny and cannot be lifted. The induration is caused by fibrosis of cutis and subcutis and is called stasis dermatosclerosis.

Atrophie Blanche

Hypopigmented painful macula are known as atrophie blanche (after Milian). It occurs almost exclusively in chronic venous stasis. It is rarely seen in lupus erythematosus, progressive sclerodermia, lymphoma, or chronic myeloic leukemia. It begins as a purpuric area with development of partial necrosis leading to white scars surrounded by teleangiectases, which upon histological examination are giant capillaries. Atrophie blanche may be regarded as the end stage of stasis dermatosclerosis.

Atrophie Blanche – Pseudatrophie Blanche

White scars developing in areas of former ulceration are *not* atrophie blanche but pseudatrophie blanche. Atrophie blanche does not result from leg ulcer.

Chronic Venous Insufficiency Stage III (Fig. 15)

The main clinical feature of stage III is present or former leg ulceration, with its localization almost always at the medial malleolus. In 20% of cases other areas of the lower leg are afflicted. The base of the ulcer is at times yellow or white. Appearance of black necrotic crusts implicates additional impairment of arterial perfusion.

Hemodynamic Changes in Venous Leg Ulcer

During rest, peripheral venous pressure is equivalent to hydrostatic pressure. This is true for both healthy persons and patients with venous insufficiency. As soon as the calf muscles are exercised, for example, during walking, incompetent veins cause additional venous hypertension, leading to reflux into superficial veins via communicating veins. The reason for microcirculatory impairment is not persisting venous occlusion but regurgitant blood flow within the veins and venoles.
In photoplethysmography it can be shown that intermittent retrograde flow reaches venoles in diseased skin but not in healthy surrounding skin.

Venous Reflux Plays the Decisive Role

Reflux, the consequence of incompetent valves, is diagnosed by directional Doppler ultrasound or ascending phlebography. It results in an incomplete decline of venous pressure during muscular exercise, whereas healthy individuals with correctly functioning muscular pumps show a significant decrease in venous pressure.

Fig. 14.
Chronic venous
insufficiency
stage II,
with corona
phlebectatica
paraplantaris,
dermite ocre,
cranial
"blow-outs", and
atrophie blanche

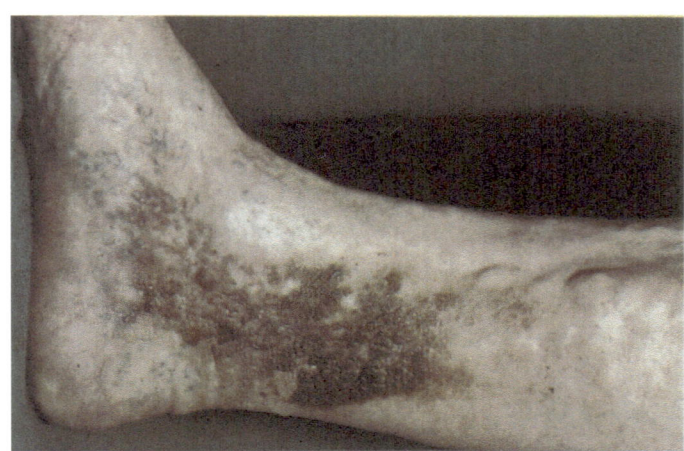

Fig. 15.
Ulcus cruris
venosum,
with cell detritus
and fibrin

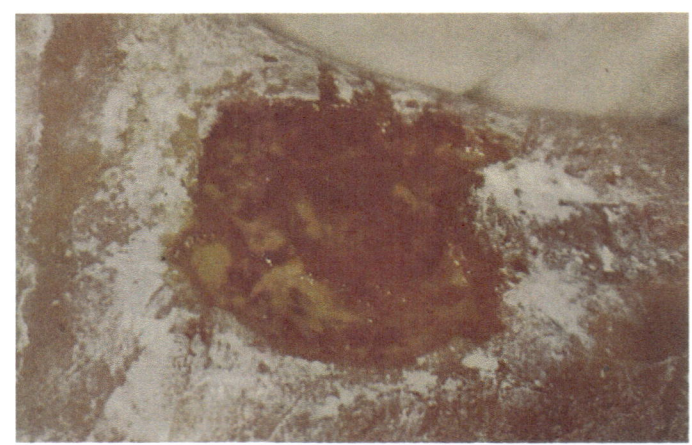

Transient Venous Hypertension

The incomplete decrease in venous pressure in patients with insufficient valves results from transient venous hypertension. Normally, pressure relief is achieved through compression by contraction of the calf muscles, which forces the blood upward while venous valves prevent retrograde flow. In patients with chronic venous insufficiency this mechanism is impaired. Therefore their mean venous pressure is increased. Such chronic venous hypertension is the main pathophysiological source of all clinical manifestations seen on the lower leg in chronic venous insufficiency. Hemodynamic conditions causing chronic venous insufficiency are very well known, but their consequences for the microcirculation and effects on the surrounding interstitial space remain to be discovered. There are presently various hypotheses concerning how chronic venous insufficiency leads to skin damage and particularly to venous leg ulcer.

Controversial Hypotheses on Venous Ulcer Pathogenesis

Numerous hypotheses have been suggested concerning the pathogenesis of ulcer formation, most of them based on clinical criteria:

Hypotheses of chronic venous ulcer pathogenesis

Stasis of venous blood	Homanns 1917
Arteriovenous shunts	Pratt 1949
Pericapillary microedema	Fagrell 1982
Pericapillary fibrin cuff	Browse 1982
Defect in fibrinolysis	Wolfe 1979
Lymphatic insufficiency	Isenring 1982
Microthrombi	Franzeck 1983
Leukocyte trapping	Thomas 1988
Overproduction of fibrosis	Leu 1980
Iron overloaded skin	Ackermann 1988

Stasis Theory

In 1917 Homanns proposed that venous stasis in dilated veins leads to tissue anoxia and subsequently to leg ulcer formation. This theory has not been confirmed, and it is no longer regarded as plausible.

Arteriovenous Shunts

In 1929 Blalock found oxygen concentration in the femoral vein of patients with chronic venous insufficiency to be higher than that in healthy individuals. Later, Holling (1938), Fontaine (1957), and Blumhoff (1976) confirmed this observation. In 1949 Pratt published the hypothesis of arteriovenous shunts below the skin causing hypoxia in the overlying cutis layer. This theory has been reinforced several times by various authors, but the existence of arteriovenous shunts was never verified.

Pericapillary Microedema

The abnormally high capillary pressure seen in chronic venous insufficiency dilates capillaries with time. Fagrell reported a pericapillary halolike formation which he ascribed to extravasation of red cells and subsequent hemosiderin deposition. According to his hypothesis, physiological metabolism and nutritional support of the skin is blocked.

Pericapillary Fibrin Cuff (Fig. 16)

In 1982 Browse proposed his model of the perivascular fibrin cuff formation: venous hypertension results in growth of dermal capillaries within the superficial cutaneous vascular plexus. Junctions between endothelial cells become wider, which he termed "endothelial stretched pore phenomenon." Increased permeability for large molecular substances such as albumine, and fibrinogen leads to loss of fluid from the bloodstream into extracellular spaces. Fibrin is of particular concern as it may form insoluble complexes after penetrating the vessel wall. These complexes enclose capillaries in a cufflike manner, consequently blocking oxygen diffusion. Local hypoxia results in the clinical features of dermatosclerosis and is responsible for cell death and ultimately ulceration. In positron emission tomography signs of oxygen diffusion blockage have been found in chronic venous insufficiency.

Defect in Fibrinolysis

Wolfe reported that patients suffering from recurrent thrombophlebitis or stasis dermatitis have reduced blood and tissue fibrinolysis activity. This impairs perivascular fibrin degradation, adding to fibrin cuff formation (see above).

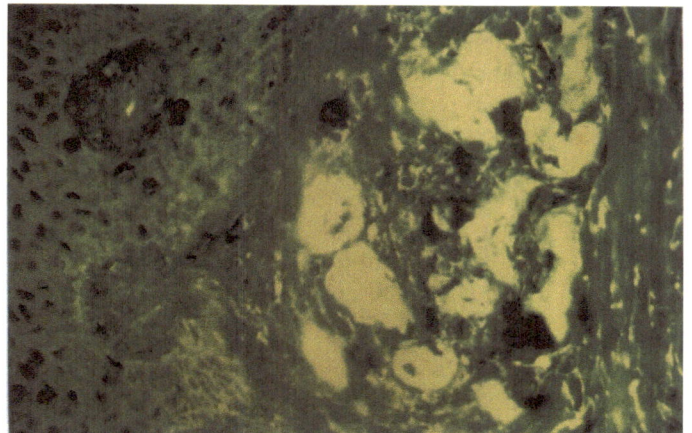

Fig. 16.
Subepidermal
pericapillary fibrin
cuff at the margin
of a leg ulcer.
Immuno-
fluorescence
staining, x 150

His findings suggest that defects of the extrinsic fibrinolysis system play a role in various forms of chronic venous insufficiency.

Earlier, in 1959, Todd reported walls of peripheral veins to contain fibrinolysis activating substances. As tissue plasminogen activators, these are part of the extrinsic fibrinolysis activating system. Todd incubated frozen vein sections on fibrin-coated plates at 37°C and recorded the amount of fibrinolysis seen as halos in the plate. Browse used Todd's method to determine tissue fibrinolysis activity at various sites of the superficial vein system. He found that the wall of the saphenous vein (above the malleolus) of stasis dermatosclerosis patients shows significantly lower fibrinolysis capacity than that of healthy persons or patients with uncomplicated varicosis of the greater saphenous vein. He concluded that either the vessel wall is deficient of fibrinolysis activators, or the consumption of these factors is increased in dermatosclerosis patients. Another indirect indication for fibrinolytic impairment is diminished ^{125}I-labeled fibrinogen clearance in extremities of patients suffering from dermatosclerosis due to chronic venous insufficiency.

Lymphatic Insufficiency

Current knowledge on lymphatic supply and drainage of the skin is limited. The lymphatic system is definitely involved in the pathophysiological processes; the extravasated fibrinogen is absorbed by lymphatic vessels and transported to the circulation. In a dog experiment it has been shown by ligature of the femoral vein that the fibrinogen content of the lymph significantly increases as a consequence of acute venous hypertension. In more severe stages of chronic venous insufficiency microlymphangiopathy has been observed in the skin of the lower leg with inadequate function of initial lymphatic drainage. Furthermore, there is a marked reduction in lymph transport in the greater lymph vessels located in the subfascial space next to the main veins. As a consequence, protein accumulates within the interstitial space of the lower leg. Lymphatic incompetence may therefore be an additional factor impairing fibrinogen elimination, however, enhancing its perivascular polymerization.

Capillary Occlusion by Microthrombi
(Fig. 17)

Fibrin clots have repeatedly been found upon histological examination of venoles and capillaries in venous leg ulcers. By fluorescence videomicroscopy Franzeck showed considerable rarification of vessels in the skin of the lower leg of patients suffering from chronic venous insufficiency. Skin maintained from an area of atrophie blanche contained avascular zones and fresh microthrombi. Franzeck drew the conclusion, that decreased perfusion by microthrombi is the crucial element in pathogenesis of leg ulcers. Microthrombi cause capillary necrosis, which leads to vessel rarification, contributing to decreased transcutaneous oxygen partial pressure.

Capillary Occlusion by Leukocytes

Another hypothesis ascribes venous ulcer pathogenesis to impaired leukocyte rheology. Microfiltration, which analyzes leukocyte flow, was performed in patients with peripheral arterial occlusive disease stage IV. Blood was drawn from ischemic legs just before amputation. Obtained leukocytes were difficult to filter, whereas after amputation leukocytes from the same leg showed improved filtration.

Moyses compared blood counts (white blood cells, red blood cells, and hematocrit) from the saphenous vein after 30 min of orthostasis with legs elevated. He found that in the group in whom the legs were not elevated leukocyte counts were lower than in the other group. His conclusion was that white blood cells adhere to a greater extent within the microcirculation of the lowered extremities; this is the case when the patient stands in an upright position.

This phenomenon was examined by Thomas in patients with postthrombotic syndrome using the same technique. His findings were consistent with those of Moyses. In detail, he reported increased adherence of granulocytes to the capillary endothelium in orthostatic legs, which was reversible when the leg was lifted to a horizontal position. In the case of decreased perfusion pressure such as in chronic venous insufficiency granulocytes are activated and stick to the vessel wall, thus hindering capillary circulation and leading to tissue hypoxia. Secondly, activated granulocytes release mediators damaging endothelial cells and increasing capillary permeability.

Increased Fibrosis

In the course of chronic venous insufficiency fibrosis advances continuously and, in atrophie blanche – the extreme version of stasis dermatitis – reduces blood flow in nutritive capillaries zero. Fibrosis extends to cutis and subcutis but also to the crural fascia. Consequently, muscles of the lower leg become atrophic; in computer tomography fatty tissue surrounding the achilles tendon seems to be thickened. Often solid scar layers (Fig. 18) are found in leg ulcers. Even periosteal ossifications (Fig. 19) have repeatedly been reported in chronic venous insufficiency.

Tissue Damage Secondary to Iron Deposition

In a spectrometric study Ackermann investigated the iron content of skin of the lower leg. The author found extremely high iron concentrations in chronic venous insufficiency, suggesting that interstitial hemosiderin deposition releases radicals, specifically oxygen radicals. These cause tissue damage and in the long run ulcer formation.

3.2.4 Diagnosis

In most patients characteristic complaints and features allow the physician to readily classify the origin of the leg ulcer. In some complicated cases very specific diagnostic evaluation by a specialist is needed to the determine cause or the adequate treatment program.

Most Important Is Ulcer History

Comprehensive history and physical examination of the ulcer patient are necessary steps in establishing a proper

Fig. 17.
Fibrin thrombus
filling capillary
lumen in venous
leg ulcer

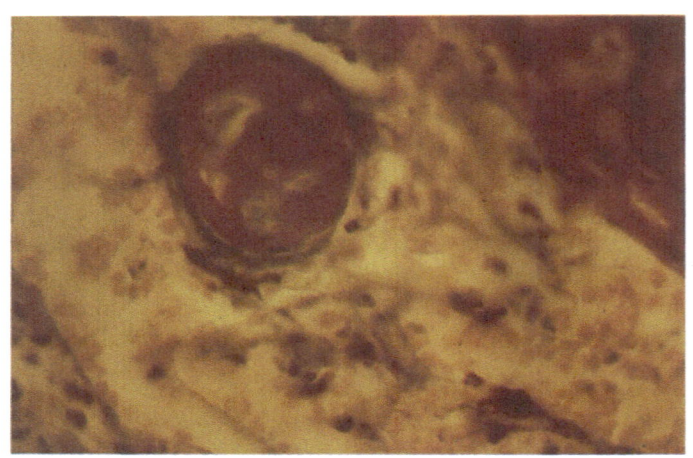

Fig. 18.
Solid scar layer
of an advanced
venous leg ulcer
with fibrin scab
on surface

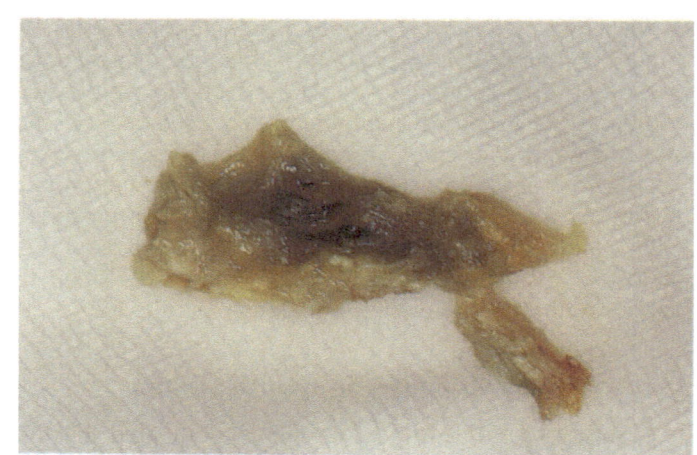

Fig. 19.
Ossification within
a chronic leg ulcer

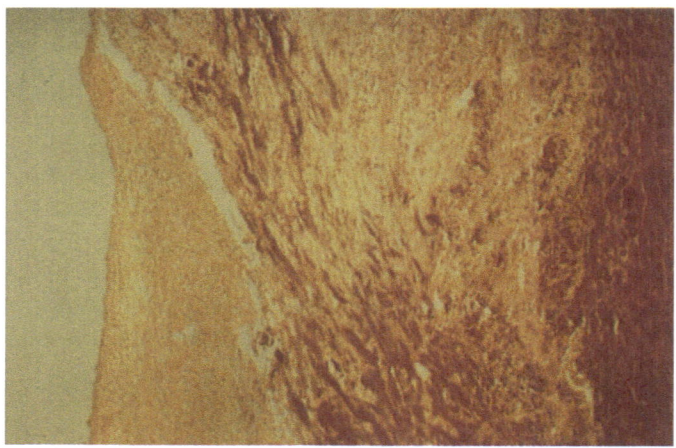

diagnosis. Determining the cause of ulcer formation is of the same importance as identifying accompanying diseases because these inevitably influence treatment and prognosis.

In Many Cases Doppler Is a Sufficient Test

Anatomic localization and stage of epifascial venous insufficiency and obstructions can generally be determined by physical examination and repeated continuous-wave Doppler tests (simple bidirectional pocket apparatus is sufficient). Doppler measurement of ankle blood pressure provides data on possible arterial disease. Arterial flow is checked by placing the blood pressure cuff around the distal lower leg and measuring the blood pressure, for example, of the dorsal pedal artery.

Cave: Diabetics

In diabetic patients ankle blood pressure measurements are not reliable. Alternative tests are measurement of toe blood pressure or digital plethysmography. Diagnosis of venous insufficiency should combine functional and anatomic evaluation. It is useful in some cases to perform diagnostic tests using a narrow tourniquet which compresses superficial veins.

Plebography Is Not Mandatory

Invasive tests such as phlebography are not necessary unless surgical intervention is contemplated. Phlebography may also be carried out in severe chronic or recurrent ulcer disease to facilitate evaluation.

Diagnosis of chronic leg ulcer

Ultrasound Doppler	+++
Photoplethysmography	+++
Duplex ultrasound	++
Phlebography	+

+++	Mandatory
++	Advisable, if available
+	In exceptional cases required

3.2.5 Compression Treatment (Fig. 20)

The basic treatment of chronic leg ulcer should accord with a physician's general rules of patient management, taking the personal needs of the patient into account and not concentrating merely on the wound. The patient's life style, mobility, job, adiposity, and accompanying diseases are substantial aspects of treatment regimens.

Compression-Pressure Gradient Must Be Maintained

Bandages must be applied in such a way that the pressure gradient is greater around the ankle and below the knee.

Only Competent Application Is Beneficial

Compression bandages may be useless or even worsen the situation if inadequately applied. Well-trained professional staff should be the only persons administering compression bandages. Arterial occlusive disease is not regarded as an absolute contraindication for the use of compression bandages as long as compression is moderate during rest.

Fig. 20.
Correctly applied compression bandage

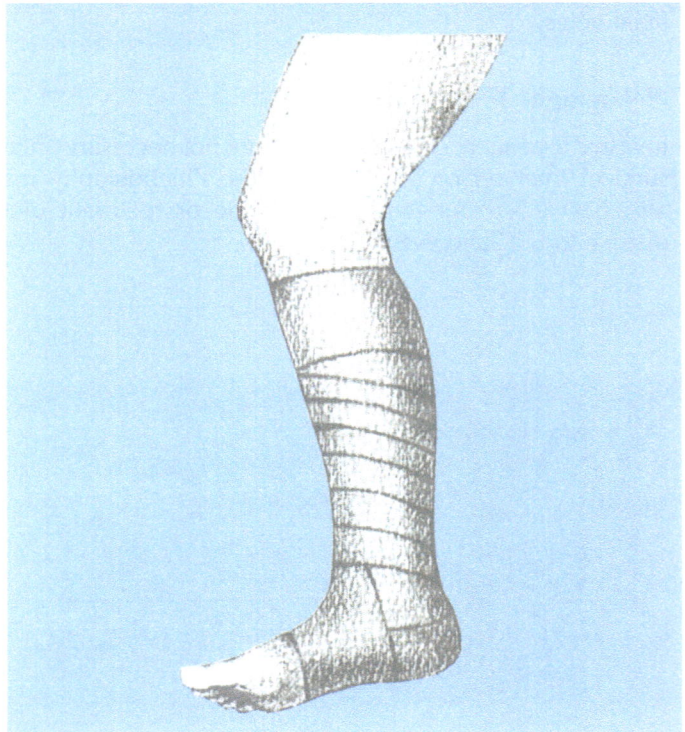

Before starting this treatment ankle blood pressure must be determined by Doppler: patients with values below 70 – 80 mmHg must be treated very carefully and frequently controlled.

Selection of Compression Bandage

The pressure dressing is selected according to therapeutic intention and activity of the patient: In standing position pressure must be higher than 60 mmHg to effectively compress deep veins of the leg. It should be noticed that compression pressure varies with different activities and positions (standing, lying) of the individual.

How Does the Compression Bandage Work?

Pressure exerted by elastic bandages is proportional to bandage tension and inversely proportional to the diameter of the skin surface. According to the rule of Laplace compression is more intense on a markedly convex than on a completely rounded surface (upper leg). Adipose patients will obtain stronger compression than lean persons with thin legs. Selective compression is achieved by intensifying pressure e.g. by putting a foam sheath on top of the leg ulcer.

Rest Versus Exercise Pressure

Pressure during rest: The stretched bandage tends to regain its original size. This generates pressure affecting underlying tissue.

Pressure during exercise: This is created by the resistance the bandage exerts against muscle contraction which results in an increased leg volume. Amplified pressure during muscle activity intermittently compresses the deep venous system.

Important: Bandage Type

Pressure impact varies with the selected bandage. Barely stretchable bandages expand very little, resisting the increased volume during muscle contraction. However, stretchable bandages permanently occlude superficial veins as pressure remains approximately the same during rest and exercise.

Effects of Compression

Elastic compression bandages cause reduced venous diameters. This diminishes venous reflux while venous flow and subfascial lymphatic transport capacity are enhanced. Consequently, interstitial pressure increases, which leads to edema resorption. Fibrinolytic activity may be enhanced.

Material

Elastic bandages and stockings are made from various materials: cotton, polyamide, polyurethane, india rubber, and others.

Elasticity of the Bandage

Bandages are categorized according to their stretchability. Barely flexible bandages (stretching capacity: less than 70% of the original size), moderately flexible bandages (70% – 140%), and highly flexible bandages (more than 140%). Bandages of 8 cm width are used for feet and those of 10–12 cm for lower and upper leg.

Application of Pressure Dressings

It is mandatory to apply the bandage in the morning, if possible before getting up, to anticipate orthograde edema formation. The foot should be kept at a right ankle when applying the bandage from distal to proximal with progressively diminishing pressure. Maximal pressure must be obtained at the ankle and foot region while the lower leg should be moderately compressed. Constant dressing pressure also guarantees a pressure gradient as diameters vary from ankle to the upper leg.

Unna's Paste Dressing

Due to its low elasticity Unna's paste dressing is hardly affected by muscle movement and therefore ensures a particular effect on the deep venous system. At the start of therapy dressings must be changed every few days (edema resorption), later on less frequently (1–2 weeks).

3.2.6 Drug Therapy

Systemic treatment of leg ulcer with the above drugs constitutes an adjuvant, supporting compression therapy. Various substances are used, such as venous tone strengthening dihydroergotamine, edema-protective flavonoids, horse chestnut extracts, tribenoside and benzarone, prostaglandins, and pentoxifylline.

Venous Tone Stimulation

Stimulation of venous tone by the use of dihydroergotamine has an effect upon the entire venous system to some extent. It may lead to an increase in central venous pressure followed by reduced venous return from the ulcer area if the dose is too high. To avoid this, medication is started with a maintenance dose (not a high initial dose) and is gradually increased. About 90 % saturation is achieved after 4 days, with a biological half-life of 1 day.

Under this therapy an increased tone of the large veins has been reported, but not of the venoles, which would result in increased postcapillary resistance and subsequently edema formation.

Edema Prophylaxis

The set of edema-protective drugs includes substances which prevent or retard edema formation. Loss of protein-rich fluid into interstitial space is decreased by a protective effect on the endothelium. In spite of their nontoxic character the flavonoids troxerutine, O-(ß-hydroxyethyl)-rutin, rutin-aescinate, and diosmine should not be used in high doses because of a diminished therapeutic effect with increasing doses.

Horse chestnut extracts or purified aescine have high interface activity and thus adhere in a prolonged manner to the affected area, which is the endothelium. They may be administered orally in the form of saponins and preferably with meals due to the common gastric irritations.

Tribenoside is a synthetic glycoside which in addition to edema prophylaxis shows anti-inflammatory properties. Occasionally it provokes skin exanthema.

A further property of benzarone in addition to protection from edema is fibrinolytic activity restricted to the intravascular space since the agent does not escape the blood stream. Side effects are moderate, sometimes seen as gastric and skin irritations. Coumarin has proven successful experimentally as an oxygen radical inhibitor and may reduce destructive leukocyte effects on the endothelium.

Systemic therapy of leg ulcer may also be performed by using prostaglandin E_1, which may be helpful when administered intra-arterially or intravenously in peripheral arterial perfusion impairment. The controversy over the pathogenesis of chronic venous leg ulcer led to the development of various adjuvant drug therapies, the effectiveness of which must in part still be proven by clinical trials. Considering pericapilllary fibrin cuffs as a consequence of impaired fibrinolysis and therefore as a main etiological factor of ulcer formation, the effect of prostaglandin E_1 has been examined in several studies. Since prostaglandin E_1 is a known stimulant of fibrinolysis and inhibitor of granulocyte oxygen radical formation, two main pathogenic components of venous ulcer disease can be influenced beneficially by prostaglandin E_1: impairment of fibrinolysis and granulocyte activation.

According to recently published data, ulcer healing is enhanced during intravenous prostaglandin E_1 infusion. Thrombophlebitic vein irritation may cause increased pain in the ulcer or an atrophie blanche area, which would certainly terminate such treatment.

Pentoxifylline is a hemorrheological agent which improves flow quality and shape flexibility of erythrocytes, stimulates fibrinolysis, hinders platelet aggregation and inhibits activation and adhesion of neutrophilic granulocytes to the endothelium. These findings led to the Anglo-Irish leg ulcer study, which found the healing rate significantly improved in the pentoxyfilline-treated group compared to compression therapy or local therapy only. These results must be reproduced in large clinical trials. A further approach is intravenous or retrograde infusion (in the manner of Bier's vein anesthesia) of urokinase. Initial studies reveal increased transcutaneous oxygen concentration at the ulcer rim under urokinase therapy.

Presently, the definite role of adjuvant therapy in venous leg ulcer disease has not yet been determined. At least it can be stated that due to the continuously growing knowledge on pathogenesis very attractive approaches have been developed which may one day add to classical compression therapy.

3.2.7 Surgical Intervention

Surgical management of chronic venous leg ulcer includes correction of dysfunction of the venous system (crossectomy, stripping), skin grafts, ulcer excision, endoscopic perforating vein dissection with or without fasciotomy, paratibial fasciotomy, and deep vein surgery.

Surgical management of chronic venous leg ulcer

Surgical procedures on the vascular system:
Crossectomy with or without stripping
Perforans ligature
Perforans discission
Endoscopic perforans discission
Transplantation and reconstruction of venous valves
Bypass operation

Transplants:
Reverdin's graft
Punch biopsies
Mesh graft
Keratinocyte culture
Skin equivalents

Surgical procedures for leg ulcer:
Ulcer excision
Fascia operation
Paratibial fasciotomy

Goals of Surgical Therapy

Corrections of the venous system to improve transitory venous hypertension, which removes the ulcer source, is one aim of surgical therapy. Secondly, ulcer healing may be promoted when covered with a skin graft. Nevertheless, compression therapy is of additional help before and after any surgical intervention.

Vein Surgery

Surgical management of venous leg ulcer is complex and involves different techniques. Surgery should always be applied in addition to other treatment measures including compression therapy, especially during the postoperative course.

Uncomplicated Surgical Intervention Should Be Tried First

Prior to surgery of the deep veins corrective intervention of incompetent superficial and/or perforating veins should be performed to avoid complicated procedures. Ligature of insufficient perforating veins is carried out if their localization is precisely defined; functional impairment may be demonstrated by Doppler and photoplethysmography.

3.2.7.1 Reverdin's Graft

Satisfying results using Reverdin's graft have been reported by Dutch authors. After local anesthesia, the corium and epidermal layer of the upper leg skin are lifted with a pointed needle and then transposed to the cleaned, granulating ulcer site. The miniflaps have an approximate diameter of 4 mm and reach the middle of the corium in depth.

3.2.7.2 Punch Biopsies (Fig. 21)

Punch biopsies are equivalent to full thickness skin grafts. Punchs of 6 mm in diameter are taken from healthy skin and placed on the wound with 5 mm distance from one another. The donor sites are closed by suture.

3.2.7.3 Mesh Graft (Fig. 22)

A conditioned wound base is mandatory for successful mesh grafting. It is a very elegant method since drainage of wound exsudate is ensured. Furthermore, topical treatment of the ulcer base may be continued after transplantation.

3.2.7.4 Paratibial Fasciotomy (Fig. 23)

Paratibial fasciotomy is quite the opposite of endoscopic dissection of perforating veins, which corrects impaired hemodynamics by removal of incompetent perforating veins. By paratibial fasciotomy a wide space is created, improving disturbed communication between the superficial and deep vein systems. Besides, the in-growth of new capillaries from the subfascial space into the liposclerotic superficial space is enhanced.

Technique

Following incision of the fascia just next to the tibia down to the medial malleolus, the fascia is dissected up to the medial condyle. Posterior perforating veins are subfascially ligated and dissected. Postoperative antibiotic prophylaxis is often required to avoid subfascial infections. Success rate of paratibial fasciotomy is very high: More than 90% of venous leg ulcers recover after being treated in such a way. The decision to perform fasciotomy, nevertheless, should only be made in selected cases. Operation is only indicated after consequent conservative therapy has failed.

3.2.7.5 Alternative Operative Procedures

Vein valve transplants, valve plasties and venous transposition procedures are still in a stage of development. These operations should be performed only at specialized medical centers in the form of well-organized clinical trials. The first operations in carefully selected patients bearing optimal anatomical conditions had disappointing results: hemodynamic parameters rarely improved postoperatively.

Fig. 21.
Punch biopsies on
ulcus cruris

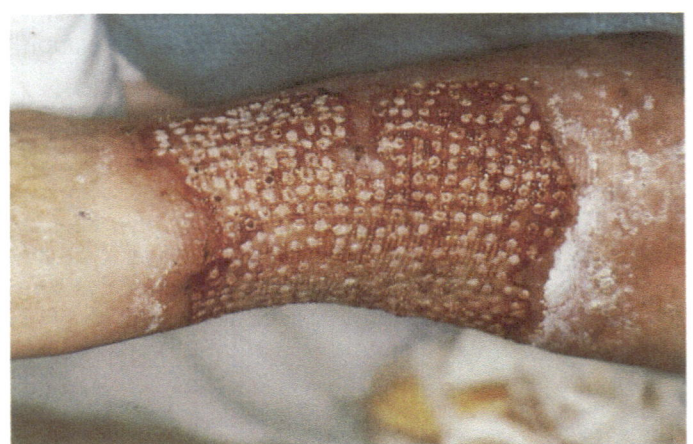

Fig. 22.
Mesh graft on
ulcus cruris

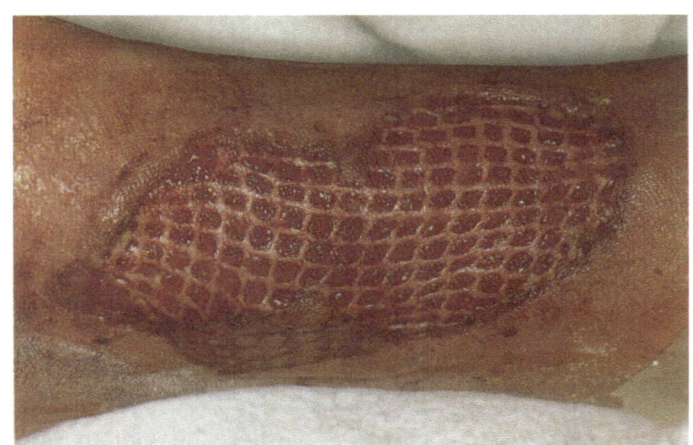

Fig. 23.
Paratibial
fasciotomy

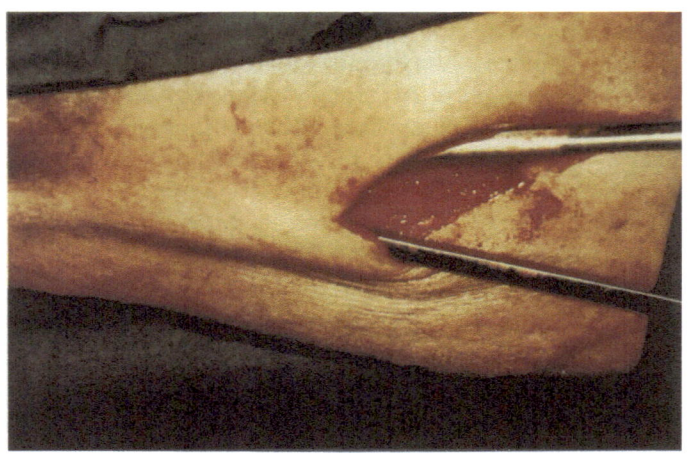

3.3 Ischemic Ulcers of the Lower Extremities

3.3.1 Pathogenesis and Clinical Features

Quite often ischemic leg ulcer (ulcus cruris arteriosum, arterial crural ulcer), which is defined as ulcer formation due to arterial vascular disease, is not recognized. It must always be considered in the differential diagnosis of leg ulcer, since its treatment is quite different from that of venous leg ulcer.

Ulcers in Arteriosclerosis Obliterans

The most common reason for arterial ulcer disease of the lower extremity is arteriosclerosis of large and medium-sized arteries followed by ischemia. The morphological causes of ischemia are lesions and changes in the intimal surface possibly leading to stenosis and complete occlusion of the involved vessel. Second to this, circulation is impaired, its severity being determined both by the extent of stenosis and by the number of collateral vessels. Collateral circulation which originates from preformed vessels may compensate for complete occlusion in many cases. A prime example is the very common obliteration of the superficial femoral artery, which is fully compensated by the formation of wide-lumen collaterals from the deep femoral artery, (perforating segments). Known risk factors are cigarette smoking, hyperlipidemia, hypertension, diabetes mellitus, adiposity, and gout. According to epidemiological studies, cigarette smoking is the major risk. Individuals bearing one additional risk factor run a twofold enhanced risk, and those with two additional risk factors live with an 11-fold enhanced risk of developing arterial obliteration of the extremities compared to persons with no risk factors at all.

Clinical Characteristics (Fig. 24)

Most of those affected are over the age of 45. Preferred localization of ischemic ulcers are the tips of the digits, around the toe nails, the nail bed, and over bony prominences such as the first and fifth metatarsal heads, calcaneus, and malleoli. Their appearance may also result from undue pressure of shoes or develop from already existing corns (clavi). Because of this, treatment of these small defects in patients with impaired circulation should not be aggressive. An early symptom of ulceration may be dark blue to black hemorrhages on the tips of the toes.

Fig. 24a
Preferred location
of arterial ulcer

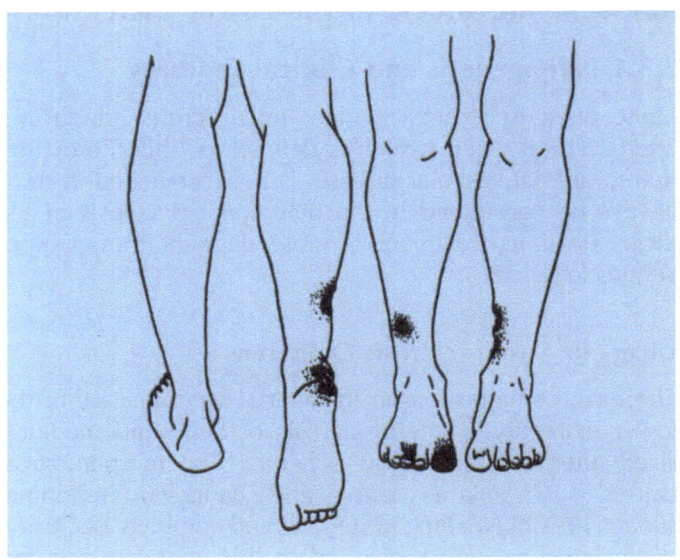

The differentiation between arterial and venous leg ulcer can be difficult since there are no definite typical localizations of arterial ulcers on the lower leg. They tend to be more commonly located on the extensor side of the lower leg (tibial margin) or at the lateral and medial malleolus. Ischemic ulcers appear to be extremely painful in contrast to the venous type. Necrotic areas and exposed tendons and bones are pathognomonic features of ischemic ulcers. Lesions are remarkably dynamic since initially they are shallow and small, gradually increasing in size. Signs of bacterial infection must be monitored carefully: hyperthermia, dolent redness, and edema of surrounding tissue may be associated with beginning phlegmonic inflammation.

Patients suffer not only from local problems but also from general symptoms of arterial occlusive disease. These may not be apparent in the initial phase of the disease. Therefore the patient must be interviewed in great detail. Arteriosclerosis obliterans is graded into four stages according to Fontaine (Table 4, p. 64). The presence and severity of arteriosclerosis obliterans can be determined by clinical examination alone: if there is no intermittent claudication with exercise a relevant stenosis imparing circulation cannot be present; the asymptomatic stage I is often missed. Depending on the particular vessel involved, severe stenosis/obliteration produces symptoms in typical locations. Three segments of localization can be differentiated:

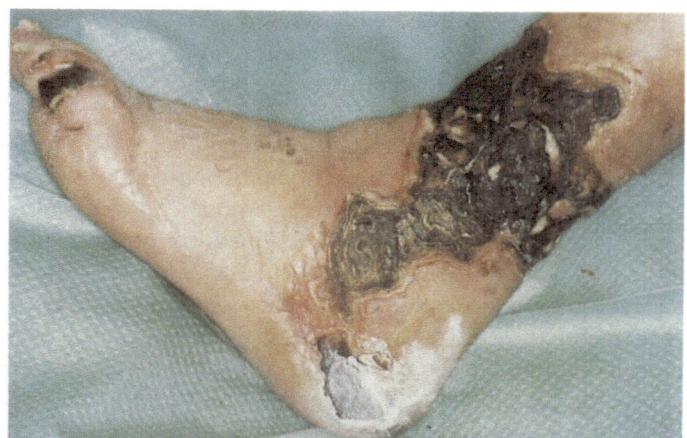

Fig. 24b.
Arterial ulcus cruris

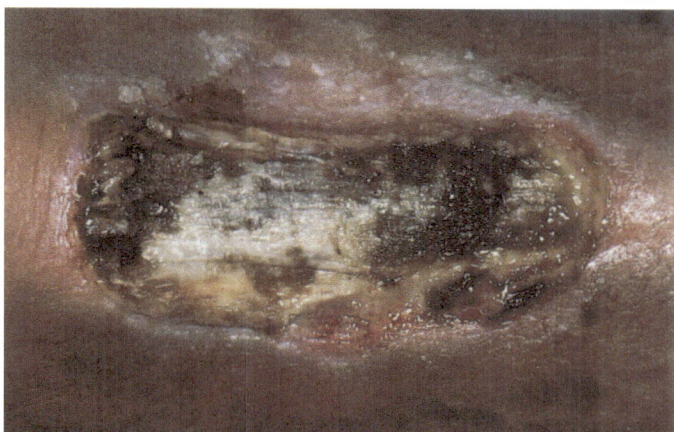

Fig. 24c.
Ulcus cruris in
the achilles tendon
region

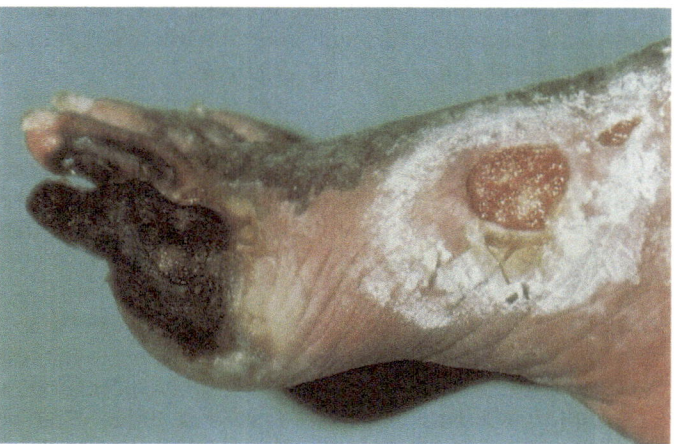

Fig. 24d.
Arteriosclerotic
gangrene

- Aortoiliac region = pelvic type
- Femoropopliteal area = upper leg type
- Infrageniculate region = lower leg type

Pain during walking or muscle exercise in general, in the foot or sole of the foot area, points to obliteration within the three arteries of the lower leg (tibial, posterior tibial, fibular) or the popliteal artery. Obliteration of the femoral artery is usually associated with aching calf muscles; Iliac or aortic obliteration is accompanied by pain in the upper leg and pelvic region. The symptom of pain during muscle work results from increased deposition of intermediate metabolic products such as lactate in muscle tissue. This forces the patient to immediately rest, which is easily and quietly done in front of shopping windows (shopping-window disease) until pain is relieved. The distance a patient is capable to walk (claudication test) is a decisive parameter in determining whether to operate.

In the advanved stages III and IV of Fontaine, arterial circulation is insufficient at rest, which is referred to as resting pain. These patients typically keep their legs dangling over the bedside in an attempt to relieve ischemic pain.

3.3.2 Diagnosis

Auscultation. Stenosis reducing the arterial lumen by more than two-thirds is heard as a systolic, pulse-synchronous turbulent murmur. For example, flow murmurs auscultated above the common femoral artery in an asymptomatic patient point to Fontaine stage I disease.

Pulse Palpation. The following arteries of the lower leg must always to be palpated: common femoral, popliteal, posterior tibial, and dorsalis pedis. It is important to know that the dorsal pedial artery is congenitally absent in 10% and may therefore be missing.

Doppler Ultrasonography. Systolic blood pressure is determined on the lying patient above the posterior tibial artery and the dorsalis pedis artery by using a blood pressure cuff and a standard Doppler ultrasound probe. The cuff is applied closely above the ankle. A whippinglike sound is characteristic for arterial pulse. Blood pressure blow 100 mmHg is regarded as pathological. A useful ratio is the comparison of ankle pressure to brachial arm pressure. A normal ankle/brachial pressure index is 1.0 or greater.

Claudication Test. A standardized test is performed on a belt ergometer (gradient: 12.5 %, speed: 3.5 km/h) to differentiate stage IIa from IIb. The patient's subjective reports should not be taken for granted.

Angiography. The indication for angiography (arterial digital subtraction angiography) is based on the above examinations. This diagnostic procedure is imperative in all patients in whom surgical reconstructive procedures are contemplated, which is the case in Fontaine stage IIb and more advanced stages. In Fontaine stage IIa angiography gives valuable information as to the site and extent of stenosis and obliteration but has no consequences at all since stage IIa is always treated conservatively.

3.3.3 Drug Therapy

There are four main substances available for drug therapy of arterial leg ulcer:

1. Pentoxifylline
Pentoxifylline influences the flow quality of blood by improving shape flexibility of the red cells. Therefore it is referred to as an hemorrheological agent. It reduces adhesion and activation of leukocytes and leads to a decreased fibrinogen plasma level.

2. Buflomedil
Buflomedil acts by enhancing erythrocyte shape flexibility and reducing platelet aggregation. In patients with Fontaine stage III or IV disease improved collateral flow has been shown under buflomedil therapy.

3. Nitrofurylhydrogenoxalate
This substance is also used in advanced stages of arterial occlusive disease. It is thought to have an antagonizing effect on serotonin and a beneficial influence on the atherosclerotic changes of the vessel wall.

4. Prostaglandin E_1
Walking distance and healing rate of ischemic ulcer improve with prostaglandin E_1 treatment when administered intravenously or intraarterially in peripheral arterial occlusive disease.

3.3.4 Surgical Therapy

For painful, therapy-resistant ischemic ulcers due to athero-sclerotic occlusion, blood flow to the extremity in question must be improved by surgical revascularization, even in Fontaine stage IIa patients when conservative management is not successful.

Iliac Segment. A well-defined stenotic lesion or obliteration may be treated primarily by dilating the vessel by percutaneous transluminal angioplasty. The initial success rate is approximately 90%; complications – mostly at the site of puncture – are seen in 3% of patients; 3 years after the procedure approximately 85% of dilated vessels are still intact.

In unilateral extended lesions endarterectomy (desob-literation) is the operation of choice. As an alternative, especially in high-risk patients, the iliacofemoral and femorofemoral cross-over bypass have proven successful. This procedure can be used only, if the contralateral common iliac artery or the external iliac artery are intact. The aorto(-biiliac)-bifemoral bypass is performed in patients with bilateral extended occlusion of the iliac artery.

Femoropopliteal Segment. Occlusion of the superficial femoral artery within the canalis adductorius is a very common finding. Isolated occlusion and nonsufficient compensation by collaterals is regarded as an indication for a femoropopliteal bypass procedure. If there is stenosis of the ostium of the profound femoral artery at the same time, a widening vein patch ("profunda-plasty") is very effective, provided that the patient exercises daily after surgery, building up fully compensating collaterals.

Infrapopliteal Segment. If the three arteries of the lower leg are involved in arterial occlusive disease, very problematic surgical intervention must be performed for of limb salvage. Femorocrural bypass on unimpaired vessels is used if distal run-off is still sufficient. In selected cases femoropedal by-passes (onto the dorsal pedis artery or posterior tibial artery) are performed. Direct desobliteration is contraindicated in this region. If reconstruction is not possible, such as among some high-risk patients, lumbar sympathectomy may be of help. With ablation of the lumbar portion of the sympathetic chain, autoregulation of vessels is interrupted which maximally dilates vessels. Among a small, defined group of patients, lumbar sympathectomy leads to favorable results in approximately 50% of those with ischemic ulceration and gangrenic lesions. In high-risk patients sympathectomy (L2 – L4) is performed by computed tomography guided puncture and ethanol infiltration interrupting the sympathetic chain.

Ulcer in Thrombangiitis Obliterans (Buerger's Disease)

Thrombangiitis obliterans is a systemic inflammatory disease affecting mainly arteries and veins, which by thrombosis obliterate medium and small arteries in a segmental fashion. In advanced stages large vessels are also involved. Veins are affected in approx. 10% of patients. Thrombangiitis obliterans develops predominantly in men between the ages of 20 and 40 years. The majority (95%) of these are smokers. While the etiology of thrombangiitis obliterans is controversial, heavy tobacco smoking is the most significant factor associated with the disease.

Clinically the occlusive arterial disease is initially distal to the popliteal artery; history or presence of superficial phlebitis is common. The first symptom to appear is claudication in the arch of the foot, sometimes in the lower leg and in the calf. Usually the patients develop ulcerations in the tips of the toe. In about 40% ischemic symptoms appear in the hands leading to ulcerations around the finger tips.

Abstinence from any form of tobacco is effective in many cases. For severely symptomatic patients with ischemic ulceration or gangrene, bypass procedure, lumbar sympathectomy, and amputation should be considered.

Ulcer in Livedo Reticularis

Livedo reticularis is an uncommon vasospastic disorder of small arteries and arterioles that may cause ulceration. The condition is characterized by mottled cyanotic "fish-net" (reticular) patterns of the skin of the involved legs and feet. The mottling is temperature dependent and becomes more intense in cooler weather. Pulse and blood pressure in the extremities are usually not impaired. While the etiology of the disorder is unknown, miscellaneous vascular diseases such as hypertension, periarteitis nodosa, disseminated lupus erythematosus and cryoglobulinemia are present occasionally. In general, ulcerations are treated locally; sympathectomy is performed only when ulcers fail to heal.

Table 4. Clinical scoring of arterial occlusive disease, adapted from Fontaine

Stage	Pathophysiology	Clinical features
I	Reduced perfusion due to single plaques of the intima wall; compensation by collateral vessels	Asymptomatic; occasionally weakness of the legs
IIa	Plaques reduce vessel diameter; Reduced functional adaption during exercise; sufficient blood flow during rest; intermittent claudication	Pain after 150 m of walking distance
IIb	As IIa, but more intense	Pain after less than 150 m of walking distance; no resting pain
III	Functionally important arteries are stenotic or obliterated; circulation is insufficient during rest	Permanent pain
IV	As III; additionally: impaired skin perfusion	Permanent pain, necrotic skin, gangrene formation

3.4 Chemical Burns

The extent of tissue damage as a direct result of exposure to a chemical is dependent upon five factors:

- pH or concentration of the agent
- Quantity of the agent
- Manner and duration of skin contact
- Extent of penetration into tissue
- Mechanism of action of the offending agent

Of greatest importance therapeutically is the duration of contact; this indicates a very simple but effective first aid measure: after removing soaked clothes, the involved area must receive early, copious lavage (tap water) for at least 15 min. Thereby the agent is diluted and skin is cooled. Water temperature should not be too cold as the patient's temperature may drop depending on the extent of the wound. Widespread burns are rinsed with large volumes of warm water.

The principal difference to thermal burns is that tissue damage progresses until the chemical agent is externally or endogenously neutralized; this can take hours or even days. Toxicity resulting from systemic absorption of the agent is a further characteristic of chemical burns.

An extensive chemical skin lesion is treated in the same manner as a third-degree thermal burn: antibacterial agents are applied topically to the wound. Furthermore, the wound should be excised and mesh grafted as soon as possible. As in thermal burn, massive edema formation may be seen within the first 24 h, followed by hypovolemic shock in full-thickness chemical burns. Therefore, the patient needs adequate volume substitution. Toxic substances resulting from degradation of the chemical agent may contribute to kidney and liver damage, which emphazises the importance of monitoring the following parameters: urine excretion and corresponding serum parameters, electrolytes, and acid-base balance. Tetanus prophylaxis must be performed.

In alkali burns corroded skin reveals colliquative necrosis, tissue destruction as a direct result of swelling and non-reactive liquefaction of the damaged area. Highly concentrated alkali fluids and caustic metallic alkali cause corrosion by binding to tissue proteins.

Important Examples

Alkali

Substance	Symptoms/organ damage	Therapy
Gasoline immersion	External damage: erythema Erythemous systemic resorption of iron and hydrocarbons may lead to: iron intoxication	Copious lavage with H_2O $\Rightarrow$ Dimercaprol, calcium
	Renal: fatty degeneration of proximal tubules Lung: surfactant degeneration, atelectasis, lipoid pneumonia CNS: edema $\Rightarrow$ coma Liver: fatty degeneration, hepatitis	Intensive care devices (e.g., artificial respiration)
Phenol	Bronze to gray skin discoloration; systemic absorption directly proportional to size of exposed area renal: direct glomerular and tubular damage, indirect damage through precipitated hemoglobin CNS: comatose state hematological: hemolysis, decreased erythropoiesis	Lavage with large volumes of H_2O (small amounts distribute the toxic agent!) Then: quick skin wipe with polyethylene or propylene glycol If necessary: intensive care Note: alkaline urine reduces precipitation of hemoglobin!
White phosphorus	Particles may burn with air contact	Involved skin must consequently be kept under water, excision under water or after rinsing with 1% copper sulfate solution $\Rightarrow$ copper phosphate formation (remove residues)
Hot tar bitumen	Chemical-thermal injury! Depth of lesion depends on the temperature of the substance, usually no systemic resorption	Primary cooling with H_2O; removal of the agent by using e.g., sorbite; tween-80 in combination with bacitracin or neosporin dissolves tar Household remedy: butter

Acids

Substance	Symptoms/organ damage	Therapy
Hydrofluoric acid	Yellow to gray skin discoloration, partly necrotic zones, extremely painful; low concentrations may lead to retarded emergence of injury: some hours later skin reveals white discoloration; progressive damage is characterized by blister and edema formation followed by penetrating necrosis; prolonged pus secretion, preferebly subungually. Systemic effects second to hypocalcemia: hepatorenal damage, bone demineralization	Lavage with H_2O along with calcium gluconate injection (controversy: unsoluble complex formation of Ca^{2+} to Fl^- anion)

Slight skin irritation: hydrocortisone cream; monitoring of plasma calcium

Severe chemical burn: parenteral administration of antibiotics and glucocorticoids |
| Nitric acid, hydrochloric acid, sulfuric acid | Gray skin coloration, severe pain; effects limited to local injury | Lavage with warm water; estimation of burn depth may be quite difficult in the beginning $\Rightarrow$ always treat as severe injury |

Three stages of alkali burn are differentiated:

Stage I   = erythema (rubefacientia)
Stage II = blister formation (vesicantia)
Stage III = scab formation (caustica)

The lesion is associated with extreme "burning" pain; full thickness tissue damage frequently leads to extensive contraction causing functional disability of nearby joints. Alkali burns are regarded as more severe insults than acid burns. The latter are characterized by coagulation necrosis secondary to protein denaturation. The acid-burned skin manifests a light yellow to white discoloration.

3.5 Burns

3.5.1 Theory

The skin has a surface of about 2 m^2 in adults and 0.25 m^2 in a newborn. It is the largest organ of the body. Its main functions are:

- Maintainance of normal body temperature
- Barrier to evaporative water loss
- Barrier to invasive infection and toxic substances
- Metabolic activity (vitamin D synthesis)
- Sensation of touch, pressure, pain

Burns are classified in degrees of injury based on the amount and depth of epidermis and dermis involved.

Burn classification adapted from Derganc (1970):

In a *first-degree burn* destruction is superficial, involving only the epidermis. The area of injury is characterized by mild swelling and erythema, which is removable using a glass spatula. Pain – the chief symptom – usually resolves after 48–72 h. The damaged epithelium peels off in small scales within 5–10 days without scarring. The most common causes of first degree burns are sunburn and brief scalding by hot liquids.

Second degree burns (partial thickness burns) involve both the epidermis and dermis and may be superficial or deep:

1. In a *superficial second-degree burn* heat injury is restricted to the epidermis and the upper third of the dermis.

By damage of microvessels permeability is increased and results in the leakage of large amounts of plasma. This fluid lifts off the injured epidermal layer which appears clinically as blister formation – the main feature of second-degree burn (Figs. 25, 26). Disrupted blisters show a light pink, moist, soft wound base. Frequently, second-degree burns are initially regarded as first-degree burns since blister formation may occur later, 12–24 h after burn. These wounds are extremely painful due to the fact that pain receptors (as well as sweat glands and hair follicles) are intact. Capillaries in the deep dermal layer are not thrombotic, which can be determined by provoking bleeding through needle puncture. Despite loss of the entire basal layer of the epidermis the wound heals in 7–14 days depending on the amount of surviving epithelial cells in skin appendages. Minimal scarring is expected to occur.

2. *Deep second-degree* or deep dermal *burn* extends into the dermal papillae, and fewer viable epidermal cells remain. Blister formation hardly occurs as the sufficiently thick dead tissue layer adheres to underlying viable dermis and may therefore not be lifted up by edema fluid. Very young and very old patients must be regarded as exceptions as their dermis is very thin. The wound surface appears red in contrast to deeper areas showing white discoloration; there is less moisture due to the severely impaired blood supply. Bleeding can be provoked only by deeply penetrating puncture. Pain is present but less intense than in superficial second-degree burn (Figs. 25, 26).

The quality of spontaneous healing depends on the ability of the deep dermal layer to regenerate. Usually dense scarring is seen after 3–4 weeks. Infection control is of great importance since wound inflammation may frequently turn second-degree into third-degree burn.

Full-thickness or *third-degree burns* involve the epidermis, dermis, and occasionally the underlying subcutaneous tissue, leaving no residual epidermal cells to reepithelialize. Characteristically, the wound shows a dry, waxy white to yellow color due to the complete absence of perfusion. In very severe burns the site of injury is of brown or black appearance, characterizing charred tissue. The elasticity of the dermis is destroyed, and the wound appears hard with increased consistency. Pain is usually absent in a full-thickness injury. Hair and finger nails can easily be removed.

Fig. 25.
Superficial second-degree burn with blister formation in an 9-year-old child

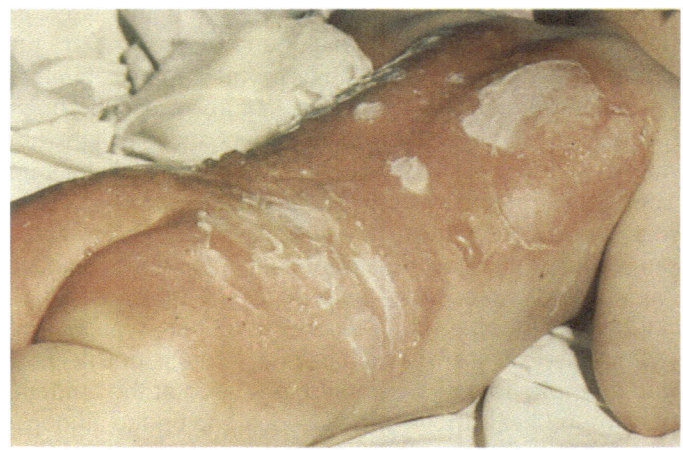

Fig. 26.
Superficial second-degree burn showing massive blister formation

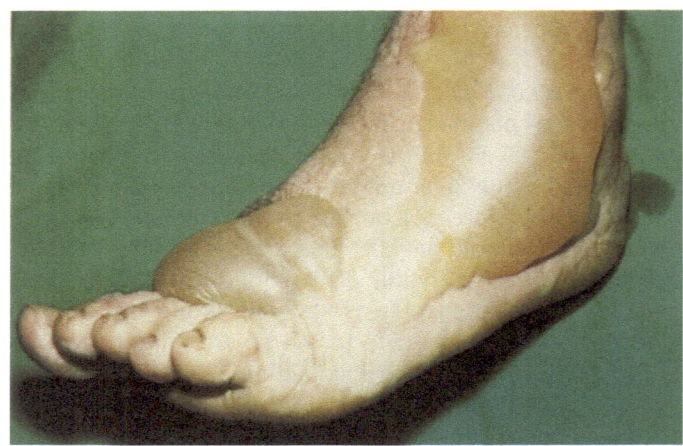

The usual causes of third-degree burns are short exposure to a very high temperature, such as flames, and prolonged contact with hot liquids. The latter also leads to hemolysis of red cells and the release of myoglobin from underlying muscle associated with red pigment deposition in the wound. This may lead to the misinterpretation of a second degree burn showing viable dermis! Therefore, it is important to emphazise that scald burns appearing in dark red color may represent a full-thickness injury.

Some authors classify charred tissue as *fourth-degree burn*. This may be used in cases when muscle tissue and possibly bone are involved. Usual causes are high-intensity flash, electricity, and prolonged contact with sources of great heat.

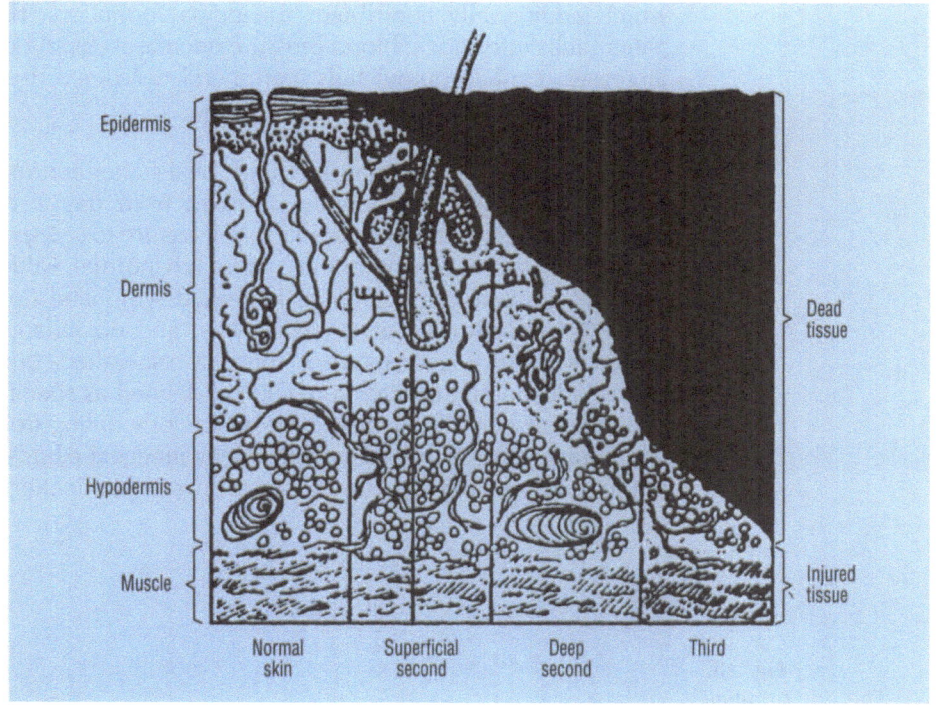

Epidermis					
Dermis					Dead tissue
Hypodermis					
Muscle					Injured tissue
	Normal skin	Superficial second	Deep second	Third	

The size of the burn is the second factor (in addition to depth) contributing to severity of thermal injury. The simplest and most readily applicable method of evaluation is the rule of "nines" (Fig. 28).

Fig. 27.
Cross-section of human skin

3.5.2 Systemic Effects of Severe Burn Injury

The presence of systemic consequences depends on the severity and the extent of thermal injury. Initially permeability is increased not in a locally restricted manner but in the entire capillary bed. This physiological change is the result of the release of various vasoactive agents, including histamine, serotonin, and kinins from mast cells. The resulting massive capillary leak is aggravated by osmotically active substances (electrolytes, low and high molecular proteins) secreted into the extracellular space.

Hypovolemic Shock

Due to above fluid shifts, plasma volume diminishes and is no longer capable of maintaining sufficient circulation. The consequences are hypoxic tissue damage and acidosis. Cell death leads to an imbalance of the sodium/potassium ratio, which additionally contributes to edema formation. The patient falls into shock: blood pressure decreases, heart rate increases, cardiac output falls, peripheral resistance rises, and urine output is reduced.

Capillary leak starts 2 h after the burn, peaks after approximately 24 h, and is gradually resorbed from day 3 on (plasma marker: urea). The capillary walls return to semipermeable function; concentrations approach normal values through compensatory osmosis; increased lymphatic flow leads to drainage of water, electrolytes, and degradation products from damaged tissue. In this phase so-called "burn toxins" (depending on literature source, defined as specific toxins or unspecific degradation products originating from denatured tissue) are resorbed which challenge the body's immune system and sometimes lead to severe intoxications.

Fig. 28.
The rule of nines helps to estimate the percentage of total body surface area burned:

each arm 9%,
each leg 2 x 9%,
front of torso
2 x 9%,
back of torso
2 x 9%,
head 9%,
each palm 1%,
genitals 1%

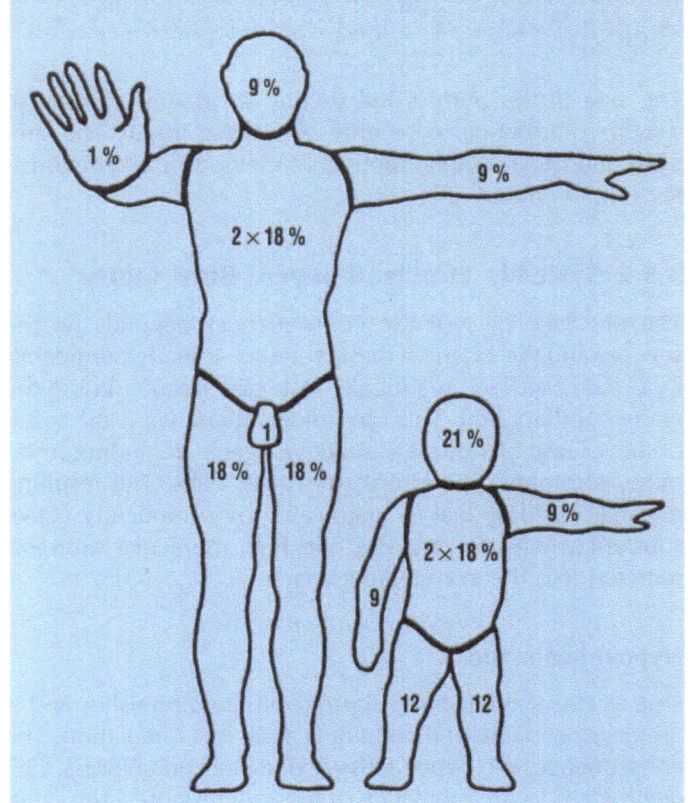

Internal Organ Damage

Internal organs are also affected by the consequences of burn injury, especially by impaired circulation and thrombosis of small vessels. Tubuli of the kidney may be damaged, which may lead to renal insufficiency; lung edema is a frequent complication due to increased alveolar capillary permeability. Inhalational injury of the lung caused by hot air, smoke, or irritant gases may lead primarily to lung edema. Furthermore, burn trauma may result in necrosis of central hepatic lobes or fatty hepatocellular degeneration. Postburn, the gastrointestinal tract is a potential source of massive bacterial invasion because of initial enteroparalysis and reduced perfusion due to edema formation within the intestinal wall. To a certain extent, intestinal dilatation leads to the translocation of physiological bacterial flora. A complication occurring in about 12 % of severely burned patients is stress ulcer (Curling's ulcer), which upon histological examination reveals hemorrhagic-necrotic changes due to impaired perfusion and reduced tissue oxygen content.

Immune System

All extensive burns affect the patient's immune system since large amounts of nonabsorbable immunoglobulins leave the intravascular space through wound exudate (3 l/m² wound/kg) or into the interstitial space secondary to increased permeability. This weakens the humoral immune system to a great extent. Cellular immunity is also impaired as seen in reduced leukocyte counts; chemotaxis and phagocytosis of these cells are often defect. In summary, the burn patient may be regarded as immunosuppressed, which makes him susceptible to infection. The injured body surface area represents an ideal medium for bacterial colonization. If topical infection control is not successful (germ concentration limit: 10^5 organisms/g tissue) the main complication is expected to occur: bacterial sepsis. To avoid this, wounds should be covered with skin transplants as early as possible to reestablish physiological bacterial defense.

3.5.3 Therapy

Immediate Management

Early treatment focuses on decreasing the potential of further local damage, which can be achieved by simple measures:

1. Flames on the victim's body or clothes must be extinguished immediately using a coat or a blanket.

2. Burned clothing must be removed rapidly as they can retain heat for considerable periods of time.

3. Use of water:
a) Immediate cooling with cold water helps to neutralize retained heat and decrease the extent of injury at depth as well as at the margins. To obtain these objectives cooling should be started even if a certain time period has relapsed between burn and first aid treatment (up to 30 min). A further benefit of cooling seems to be stabilization of skin mast cells which reduces histamine release and edema formation. A marked advantage of cooling is the decrease in pain from irritated nerve endings. The use of ice water is strictly contraindicated due to the fact that tissue hypothermia may produce additional trauma. In superficial second-degree burns with a size of less than 10 % of total body surface, cooling may be continued ad libitum to control pain. After heat neutralization of large burn wounds (more than 10 % –15 % of body surface area) cooling is no longer advisable as it has a number of disadvantages: there is increased body heat loss through the burn wound, which invariably produces shivering leading to increased oxygen consumption and calorie demand. Therefore
b) in all burns larger than 10 % –15 % of body surface area in an adult and 5 % in a child, an ambulance must be called immediately to transport the patient to a burn center. Intravenous fluid resuscitation and analgesia are started at once. The burn patient receives 4 ml/kg body weight per percent burned surface area within the first 24 h postburn.

Further indications for immediate professional medical management are burns of the head-neck area or inhalational injury since these patients may rapidly develop the need for endotracheal intubation.

4. Covering the burned area with sterile dressings.

Conservative Treatment

Perfectly sterile working conditions are of essential importance in the care of burn patients. Every one including
nursing staff, physicians, nonnursing personnel, and visitors,
must follow the infection control policy to prevent movement of organisms from dirty to clean areas or to
noninfected patients. Prophylactic measures such as wear-
ing a cap, a mask fully covering the hair, a long-sleeve
isolation gown tied in the back, and clean gloves are to be
fulfilled.

Nonsurgical wound care continues care initiated during the
immediate postburn period. Patients with large burns and
such of the head-neck area receive fluid therapy, for example, according to the following scheme. The patient's baseline body weight is measured. Fluid therapy and nutritional
supplementation are determined by changes in body weight
during hospitalization.

SCHEME: INFUSION THERAPY DAYS 1–4

Day 1

FLUID RESUSCITATION

4 ml isotonic crystalloid (e.g., lactated Ringer's injection) / kg body weight / % body surface burned (Baxter formula): one-half of the calculated volume is administered in the first 8 h posttrauma, and the remainder is given by continuous drip infusion over the next 16 h.

$\Rightarrow$ Effects:
    Fluid and sodium substitution
    Acidosis correction

Close monitoring of

1)   Diuresis (30–50 ml/h)
2)   Hematocrit (65 vol.% maximum)
3)   Mental state

ad 1) > 50 ml/h = volume overload
$\Rightarrow$ Watch for signs of pulmonary edema and brain;
    < 30 ml/h = inadequate excretion of urinary substances
$\Rightarrow$ Danger of renal damage
ad 2) Normalization is not to be expected within 24 h;
    < 45%: a) Bleeding or
           b) Volume overload must be considered.
ad 3) Reduced consciousness may appear secondary to CO or CO_2 intoxication,
    Head trauma,
    Electrical burn, or
    Beginning septicemia.

In catastrophe situations not every victim may recieve intravenous fluid resuscitation. The following simple measure has proven successful and is available almost everywhere: The burn victim must drink a volume of 15 % of his body weight, which is supplemented with one tea-spoon (approx. 4 g) of salt per liter.

Day 2

VOLUME MONITORING

ONCOTIC REABSORPTION

Fluid monitoring:
Intravenous fluid volume day 1 =
        Urine/gastric juice output
        Plus increase in body weight (edema)
        Plus evaporation (4 l/m² wound/day)
        Plus exsudation (must be calculated with this
        formula)

Intravenous fluid volume day 2 =
        Adequate urine output (approx. 2.4 l/day)
        Plus evaporation (see above)
        Plus exsudation (approx. 2/3 of day 1)
        Minus desired body weight reduction
        (50 % of edema volume)

2–3 ml lactated Ringer's solution / kg body weight / % surface area burned
+ 0.35–0.5 ml protein colloid solution (e. g., human albumin) / kg body weight / % surface area burned

$\Rightarrow$ Increase of plasma protein concentration up to 6–7 g %

Close monitoring of sodium, potassium (replace, if necessary) and plasma protein concentration

Awake patients may try peroral fluid uptake (tea, coke, sugar water)

Day 3

RETURN TO NORMAL CONDITION

OPERATION

Fluid monitoring: as day 2

Intravenous fluid volume: as day 2

Required weight reduction:
25 % of total increase in body weight
Cave: Adapt calculation of exsudation and evaporation to
        changed wound surface after skin grafting
        (donor site must be regarded as a new wound).

Electrolyte requirements:
- Potassium: replacement of 60-160 mmol is necessary
- Sodium: low serum sodium may suggest volume overload.

Day 4

NUTRITION

Baseline body weight is approached.
Due to a high metabolic rate inadequate nutrition would
lead to catabolism of fat and muscle.
⇒   Oral feeding of high caloric, protein rich nutrition,
       e.g., milk-shakes with eggs, sugar; if oral intake is
       impossible, enteral feeding by nasogastric or naso-
       jejunal tube is begun; if oral or enteral nutrition is
       inadequate due to gastrointestinal dysfunction, total
       parenteral high-caloric nutrition must be per-
       formed

Calorie and protein monitoring

Serum electrolytes check

Analgesics

Prior to cleansing and débriding of the burn wound the patient must receive sufficient analgetic medication. As pointed out above, the deeper the burn the less the pain, so that the full-thickness burn that is likely to have the greater hemodynamic instability entails the least discomfort. However, burns are usually not uniform in depth, and some second-degree burns, which are the most painful ones, are always present. Analgetic treatment should be started with small intravenous doses, 1–2 mg morphine, and increased as required relative to the hemodynamic response. Fentanyl is also an excellent analgesic because of its rapid onset of action and short half-life.

Cave: Tetanus

Tetanus prophylaxis is required (American College of Surgeons Guidelines). If there is any uncertainty about prior vaccination, or the patient is not awake, active and passive immunization must be performed.

The baseline germ concentration of the burned areas, the nasotracheal space, and the perianal area are determined by taking smears. Wounds then are washed using, for example, povidone-iodine diluted in sterile saline or water. The solution should be at room temperature or higher. It is important to gently mechanically débride the wound using gauze to remove dirt and loosen devitalized epidermis and to better determine the true depth of the burn.

First-degree burns require only symptomatic therapy, for example, a topical anesthetic spray or cream to cool the wound and reduce itching which occurs after the initial sensation of burning.

Removal of Hair (Depilation)

Second-degree burns require not only removal of devitalized tissue, disrupted blisters, and punctioning of intact blisters but also – in large burns – the removal of hair, except eyelashes and eye brows, as hair is a potential source of bacterial infection.

Edema-Associated Compression

In circular full-thickness burns of the extremities perfusion may be markedly reduced secondary to massive edema formation compressing viable tissue beneath the nonelastic burn area. Primarily, venous return is impaired, but with increasing pressure, arterial flow as well. Clinical signs include extreme pain and sensory disturbance of the extremity (appearance of cold body surface areas is fairly common in burn patients as the skin is cooled by evaporation). If there is circular injury to the neck and torso, breathing or thorax excursion during breathing may be impaired. In these cases the treatment of choice is escharotomy, which is performed by incising the burn wound eschar (anesthesia is not necessary) in a certain way to relieve pressure. In deep burns or electrical burns fasciotomy may be necessary to assess the extent of muscle necrosis and relief pressure from massive tissue edema. Although these incisions, which must later be covered with skin transplants, create additional wounding and scarring, they are of immense importance in preventing amputation.

Infection Control

A topical bacteriostatic or bactericidal chemotherapeutic agent should be applied in all second- and third-degree burns after débridement. One of the various available agents or dressings is chosen individually depending on localization and extent of the burn wound.

Povidon-iodine cream 1% is used widely due to its broad antibacterial action and its ability to penetrate the burn eschar. This preparation causes rapid desiccation, leading to formation of a dry leathery eschar. It provides reasonable protection from wound infection if applied several times a day. The disadvantages of povidone-iodine include pain upon application, systemic effects of iodine absorption, and staining of the wound, which makes clinical assessment of the wound difficult.

Aqueous silver nitrate 0.5% has a universal bacterial action, is not painful, and does not cause skin hypersensitivity. Due to its poor penetration of eschar, the dressing (thick layers of gauze) must be kept wet by the intermittent addition of more solution every 4 h between daily dressing changes. The disadvantages of aqueous silver nitrate are that these dressings heavily stain tissue, equipment, linen, and floor. Furthermore, there may be electrolyte depletion (sodium and chloride) secondary to complex formation with the silver anions (close monitoring of electrolytes is therefore very important) and methemoglobinemia with subsequent cyanosis.

Silver sulfadiazine cream is the most widely used topical agent. It contains silver anion forming complexes with a certain sulfonamide. As soon as it contacts wound fluid the two substances dissociate: the silver remains on the surface, protecting the wound from bacterial invasion; the sulfonamide penetrates the eschar acting against gram-negative organisms in a better way than against the gram-positive including *Candida*. During this treatment sodium replacement may be necessary. Approximately 4% of patients treated with silver sulfadiazine acquire hypersensitivity to sulfonamide, which leads to pain, pruritus, and rash. The agent should be applied twice daily, at a thickness of 2–3 mm on gauze bandages, which also has a cooling effect on the wound.

Mafenide acetate 10% cream has an excellent antibacterial action particularly against gram-positives and clostridia. The substance rapidly penetrates the burn eschar and is not affected by the presence of pus and serum. It is applied twice daily at a thickness of 5 mm on burned areas. Application is painful. In sulfonamide-sensitive patients mafenide treatment may result in rash. One side effect of mafenide has led to its exclusion from the European pharmaceutical market: its carbonic anhydrase inhibitory properties cause metabolic acidosis, which must be compensated for by lungs and kidneys. For patients with renal or lung function impairment, this represents a great risk.

Enzymatic Débridement

A further treatment alternative is enzymatic débridement in combination with antibiotics. Elastase or collagenase leads to lysis of necrotic areas by degrading elastin or collagen. Viable tissue remains untouched. It is important to know that this kind of treatment leads to increased exsudation during the initial postburn period, which must be compensated by intravenous fluid administration. At the same time this reduces edema, which may sometimes make escharotomy (see above) unnecessary. Collagenase-treated burn wounds show less keloid formation, scar contracture, and hypertrophic scarring.

Dressings

After the application of topical antimicrobials, wounds are covered with nonadhering grease gauze to prevent damage of the newly formed wound surface during the change of dressings. To facilitate removal the dressing should be moistened using isotonic fluid. The latter is also used to wash off the cream before the wound is examined and the chemotherapeutic agent reapplied. To avoid bacterial transmission clean or less infected areas should be treated first and rewrapped before approaching dirtier areas.

The burn wound treated with topical agents can be managed without dressings by placing the patient on cream-coated foam material and covering the wounds with a dense layer of cream. Disadvantages include a greater risk of wound desiccation, which may lead to an increase in wound depth through secondary necrosis and an increased risk of bacterial cross-contamination.

In general, all burn wounds are initially treated conservatively. Exceptions are: small but deep wounds, which are excised early on; lesions produced by electrical burn, which must be excised at once to remove toxic substances; burns in children should be excised as early as possible to avoid long-term, painful dressing changes; burns of the face or hands show better cosmetic results when early excised and grafted.

Deep second-degree and third-degree burns should be excised as soon as the circulatory and metabolic parameters of the patient are stabilized, and edema is reduced to at least 50% of the initial volume (generally day 3). Early burn wound excision reduces the potential for bacterial infection. Wound closure achieved by skin transplantation rebuilds the physiological barrier against bacterial invasion.

Temporary Skin Substitutes

There may be several reasons why early excision and wound closure cannot performed, for example, the patient's condition is unstable; other areas of the body have priority for grafting (i.e., face); the amount of skin available as donor graft is small; the wound is of varying depth and must be transformed into a homogenous wound base prior to autografting. A number of temporary skin substitutes have proven successful in maintaining a more favorable environment for wound defense mechanisms to clear surface bacteria and to prevent heat and evaporative water loss. The application of so-called "*biologic dressings*" is very reliable, which are homologous (cadaver skin) or heterologous (pigskin) skin substitutes. They should be applied to the wound after the initial removal of any loose tissue and debris. Adherence to clean wounds is usually excellent; small vessels penetrate the skin substitute within a few days. Nevertheless it must be pulled off after 5 days because of an increased risk of deep infection as bacteria may be sealed beneath the dressing forming abscesses or seroma. If this occurs, adherence of the skin substitute is usually poor. Aggressive mechanical débridement and initiation of topical antimicrobials is required. The treatment with a temporary skin substitute is continued until a granulating wound bed has formed. The skin substitute should not stay on the wound for longer than 5 days, since after 10 days rejection with subsequent perfusion impairment, autolysis, and infection would begin.

Human temporary skin substitute is generally superior to pigskin, which is more susceptible to infection. They have in common that the occlusive character of the dressings has a beneficial effect on wound secretion thus reducing protein loss. Pain is reduced, fever declines, and bacterial colonization decreases.

Synthetic skin substitutes are used in first-degree and superficial second-degree burns as an alternative to the application of topical antimicrobials. They increase the rate of epithelialization, which – as is known – is delayed when applying chemotherapeutics. A number of synthetic skin substitutes have been developed with some disadvantages such as nonflexible material reducing the patient's motility and an increased risk of infection through exsudate aggregation beneath the dressing (see also Chap. 6).

Diagnosis and Therapy of Wound Infection

Burn wounds are never sterile. Although germs are killed during the burn insult, enough bacteria remain within skin appendages and wrinkles to colonize the injured body surface. Antiseptic treatment and daily cleaning of the patient merely helps to prevent uncontrolled bacterial growth over a certain period of time (depending on the patient's condition). The assessment of bacterial contamination by taking daily wound smears – prior to the cleaning procedure – is of great importance.

There are three stages of bacterial contamination: colonization, infection, and septicemia.

The presence of bacteria only on the wound surface or in nonviable tissue, diagnosed by surface swab culture is termed *colonization*. There is neither a visible local reaction (e.g., pus) nor a systemic effect, such as leukocytosis or fever. *Infection* of the wound is the term used to indicate beginning invasion of the underlying viable tissue. The clinical diagnosis can be quite difficult as typical signs such as intermittent temperature spikes and leukocytosis are characteristically seen in the burn patient with and without wound infection. Furthermore, infected areas may be of similar appearance as colonized areas. The most reliable method of diagnosing burn wound infection is bacterial analysis of the burn wound biopsy, which must include some underlying viable subcutaneous tissue. Quantitative bacterial count and histological inspection of the biopsy is performed. The presence of 10^5 or more organisms per gram of tissue indicates infection. This can be confirmed by histology, when bacteria are seen invading viable tissue. Systemic antibiotic treatment is required. Infected wounds usually show a macerated, soft eschar and redness of surrounding tissue.

With progression, the viable tissue and its vessels are invaded, and *septicemia* develops. The patient suffers from pain due to the destruction of healthy cells. Wound biopsy reveals more than 10^5 organisms per gram of tissue. This indicates the need for systemic antibiotics.

If conservative treatment is not successful in invasive subeschar infection, tangential excision of the infected area and subsequent closure using a skin graft should be considered although there is a risk of bacterial dissemination and bleeding. The contraindication for this procedure is an unstable cardiopulmonary condition of the patient. Early surgical wound closure is the ultimately efficient way to fight bacterial infection.

Surgical Management

The primary goal of the surgical approach is to remove nonviable tissue and reconstruct the skin defect. Usually a maximum of 20 % of total body surface area can be excised at one time. If further operations are necessary, intervals between treatments should be 2–3 days, depending on blood loss and on circulatory parameters. A surgical strategy must be developed: areas which require adequate cosmetic results must be covered first; optimum planning of donor

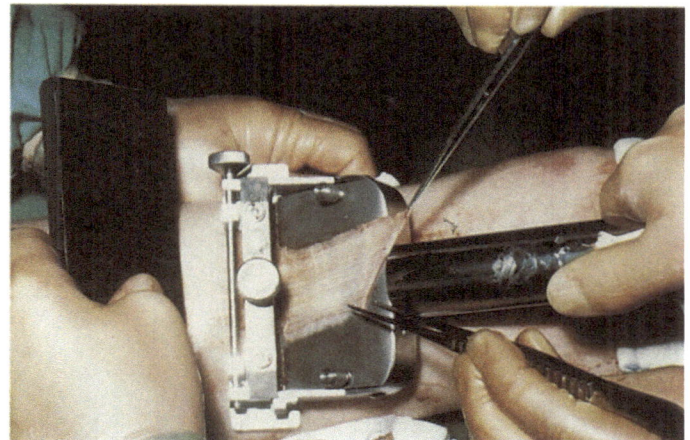

Fig. 29.
Donor skin is obtained using a dermatome

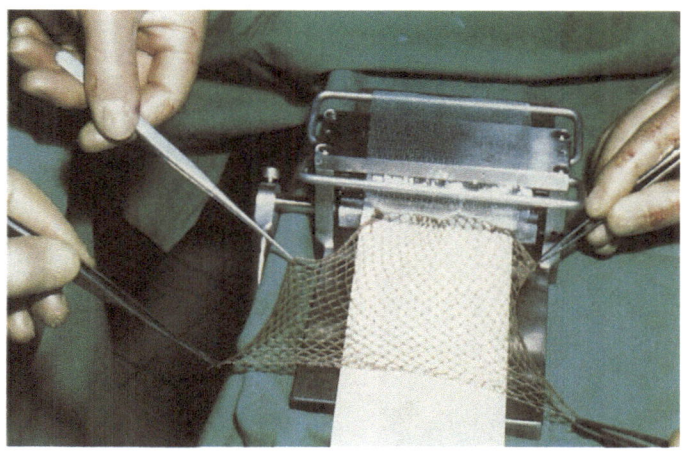

Fig. 30.
Skin is transformed into a mesh graft

Most common bacterial organisms in burn wounds

ORGANISM	WOUND APPEARANCE	ANTIMICROBIAL AGENT
Staphylococcus aureus	Yellow discoloration of necrotic tissue, nonsmelling	Bacitracin Fusidic acid Neomycin
Pseudomonas aeruginosa	Patchy green, fluorescent under UV light or blue to black necrosis, sweet smell	Mafenide Gentamicin + carbenicillin Silver sulfadiazine Povidone Iodine
ß-Hemolytic Streptococcus		Penicillin
Enterobacteriacae: Escherichia coli, Klebsiella, Proteus		Depending on resistance in culture
Candidia albicans	Black discoloration	Silver sulfadiazine

Fig. 31.
Third-degree burn

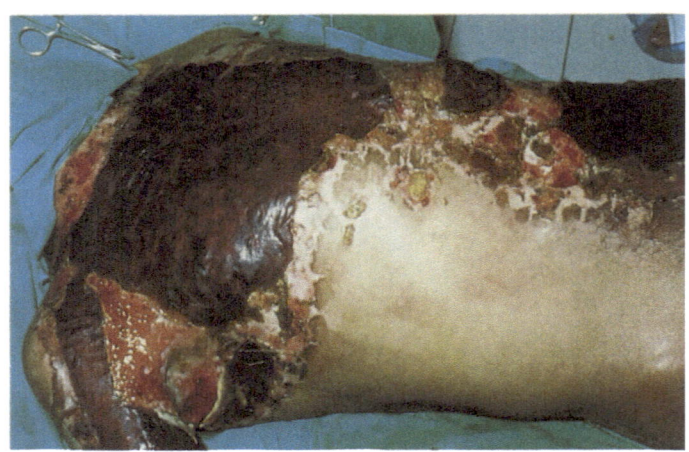

Fig. 32.
The same patient
after débridement

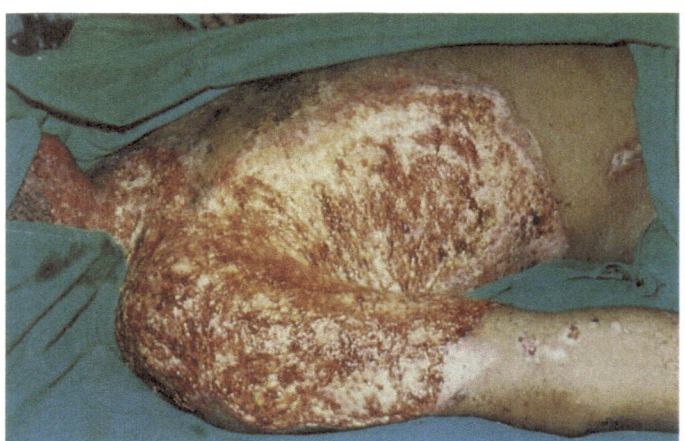

and recipient area must be performed since the thickness
and color of skin is variable.

After the hemodynamically stable patient is brought to the
operating room, all wounds to be covered during the ses-
sion are cleaned using povidone-iodine. Then a split-thickness skin graft is obtained by using a dermatome (Fig. 29) or
an electric Pagett which allows depths of 0.25–0.3 mm
(maximum: 1 mm). Thus, the epidermal and the upper third
of the dermal layer are removed, which is equivalent to a
superficial second-degree lesion healing with minimal or no
scar formation. Thighs, upper arm, abdomen, buttocks, and
calf are preferable donor sites. If these areas are injured as
well, donor sites are obtained wherever unburned skin is
available. Injection of saline beneath the dermis greatly
assists the removal of split-thickness skin from areas around
changes in contour. A number of complications may occur

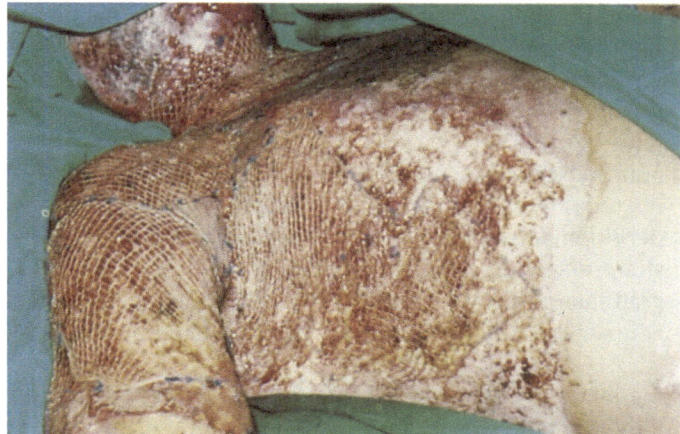

Fig. 33.
Condition after
mesh grafting

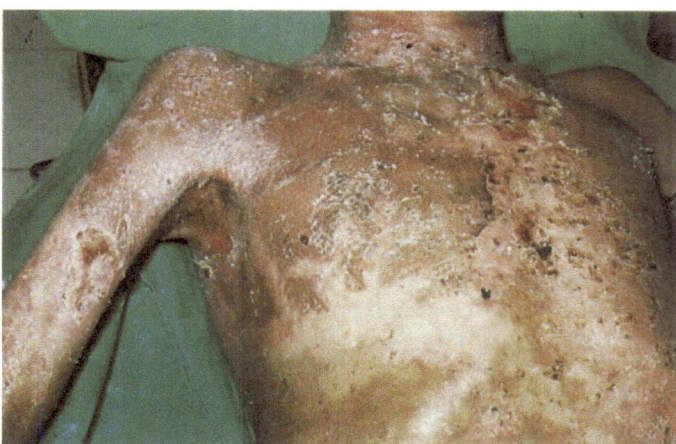

Fig. 34.
Eight weeks after
mesh grafting

at the donor site, including infection, which can result in deepening and possibly conversion of the wound to full-thickness and lead to hypertrophic scarring.

The obtained skin is kept sterile and moist until placed onto the recipient area. The donor site is covered with warm sodium-chloride soaked gauze to enhance blood coagulation. As a definite wound dressing, synthetic skin substitutes (semiocclusive dressings) have shown good results remaining on the wound for 4–5 days. Thereafter the lesions reepithelialize air-exposed.

The recipient area is then prepared. Using a scalpel or Goulian dermatome, the eschar is shaved down into viable, bleeding tissue. This process of eschar shaving is known as "sequential tangential excision." The crucial aspect of the procedure is to determine the optimal depth. Punctiform bleeding is suppressed, for example, using hydrogen peroxide soaked gauze; major bleeders are controlled with electric cautery or ligature. A saline-soaked gauze is placed on the débrided area and left while the donor skin is prepared.

Full-thickness burns and deeply charred tissue may require necrectomy down to the muscle fascia (epifascial débridement), which is performed using a combination of sharp excision, constant tension, and electric cautery. The graft take is always excellent. However, the cosmetic result is unsatisfactory due to a lack of subcutaneous tissue.

Depending on the size of the wound, the split-skin graft is either directly transferred or prepared using a mesh dermatome. Even if skin meshing is not to be performed, a number of small slits should be placed along the skin tension lines to allow efflux of any blood or plasma that collects. The skin is cut to conform to the wound shape and placed directly onto the wound surface. The graft soon adheres to the wound by fibrin exsudate, which makes sutures unnecessary in smaller wounds but requires immobilization of the area to allow graft vascularization to occur. Large grafts must be sutured, which has the disadvantage of producing bleeding, possibly lifting the graft off the wound surface. Fixing the graft by using fibrin may lead to necrosis and subsequent infection.

The method of choice to cover large burns is to perform meshing of the obtained skin graft, which increases the graft size to 1.5- to 6-fold. The skin grafts are best placed with the dermis side up on a mesh board. The mesh dermatome produces slits of variable size and distance. Best results are obtained when applying 1.5–1 meshed grafts since slit spaces completely reepithelialize. Furthermore, mesh grafting bears the advantage of draining wound exsudate through the slits. The main disadvantage is the moderate long-term cosmetic result through scar formation, which is the reason for not applying mesh grafts on the face and neck area. Mesh grafts are fixed either by applying fibrin (very expensive, limited indications) or by suturing the edges of the graft.

After grafting 1.5–1 meshed grafts are allowed to heal exposed to air (restricted to well-equiped burn centers) or, similar to wider mesh, are covered with a dressing. Grease gauze or fine mesh gauze is applied to the graft, followed by a moistened gauze layer and a dry gauze layer or bandage.

It is necessary to immobilize grafted areas. The first post-operative dressing change should be performed not earlier than 5 days later as manipulation might impair reepithelialization. If any signs of wound infection occur (e.g., pain, temperature increase, enhanced exsudation), the dressing must be removed immediately. Adequate topical antibiotic therapy is required.

3.6 Anorectal Abscesses and Anal Fistulas

3.6.1 Anorectal Abscesses

An anorectal abscess is an acute inflammatory process located within the tissue surrounding the rectum and the anal canal.

Depending on the localization, the following abscess types are distinguished:

– Perianal
– Ischiorectal
– Submucosal
– Pelvirectal (supralevator)
– Deep postanal / retrorectal

Anorectal abscesses located proximally to the levator ani muscle (supralevator abscess), such as high intermuscular, submucosal, or pelvirectal abscesses, are relatively rare, comprising less than 5 % of total anorectal abscesses. Potential penetration and invasion of further abscess cavities must always be considered during examination and therapy.

The cause of a nonspecific anorectal abscesses usually remains unclear. Commonly the condition is attributed to inflammatory disorders of the anal pits, located between anal crypts and the intersphincteric space; this is known as the cryptoglandular theory.

Specific causes include the following:

- Anal fissure
- Perianal hematoma
- Infected prolapsed hemorrhoids/infected thrombosed hemorrhoids
- Traumatic skin lesions (e.g., solid stool, scraping toilet tissue, other mechanical manipulation)
- After sclerotherapy (submucosal abscesses)

- Crohn's disease, ulcerative colitis
- Acute appendicitis or colon diverticulitis may lead to the formation of pelvirectal abcess
- Prostatitis / infection of the seminal vesicle
- Specific infections such as gonorrhea, amebiasis, actinomycosis, tuberculosis

Abscess and fistulas occur more commonly in men than in women, with a significant percentage being diabetics. The vast majority of patients develop the disease in the fourth, fifth, or sixth decade. The incidence of recurrent abscess formation is fairly high.

Smear cultures obtained from the abscess mostly present a mixed, gram-negative flora. *Escherichia coli* and streptococci are always involved. Treatment of anorectal abscesses includes identification of the organisms by culture technique, to introduce adequate antibiotic therapy.

Perianal and Ischiorectal Abscesses

The perianal (i.e., perirectal) abcess is the most common type of anorectal abcess (approximately 80% of cases), located within subcutaneous tissue around the anal verge. In many cases it is the result of infected anal crypts or originates at the site of a chronic anal fissure. When these abscesses lead to the proximal dissection or invasion of sphincteric muscles, they are referred to as intermuscular or intramuscular abscesses.

Ischiorectal abscesses are seen in about 15% of patients, located in the right or left fossa ischiorectalis. Pus is almost always present, with a volume of 60–90 ml. The two fossae may present a communicating abscess cavity through the posterior aperture of the external sphincter. This abscess type is caused mainly by cryptoglandular pus aggregation dissecting the external sphincter.

Symptoms and Diagnosis

The patient usually presents with a relatively short history of painful swelling that may be exacerbated by intestinal peristalsis, defecation, and by sitting and walking. Physical examination reveals the abscess as a swollen, erythematous area, located at the anal verge in case of an perianal abscess, larger and more laterally in case of an ischiorectal abscess. Rectal digital palpation of the perianal abscess shows fluctuance and extreme pain at contact, restricted to the anal verge. The ischiorectal abscess may be palpated along the internal wall of the anal canal. The size of the abscess is assessed using the two-digital palpation method. In large ischiorectal abscesses symptoms such as increased body temperature or chills may be seen.

Submucosal (Intersphincteric) Abscess

Submucosal abscesses are found mostly either within the lower part of the rectum or cranially to the rectoanal border. The condition arises from an infected crypt and dissects into the intersphincteric plane. It is a rare type of anorectal abscess, seen in 4% of patients.

Symptoms and Diagnosis

The symptoms are rather moderate. The patient complains of rectal discomfort, exacerbating during defecation, and possibly of a rise in temperature. Physical examination may be unrevealing; however, the abscess presents at digital palpation of the rectum as a tender submucosal mass possibly protruding well into the lumen.

Pelvirectal (Supralevator) Abscess

Pelvirectal abscess – some authors refer to this as supralevator abscess – is relatively rare, comprising less than 1% of anorectal abscesses, located cranially to the fascia of the levator ani muscle on the left or right hand side. The following anatomic structures surround the abscess cavity: cranial = peritoneum, lateral = ligaments, posterior = rectum, distal = levator ani muscle, anterior = urinary bladder and – depending on sex – urethra, prostata, and seminal vesicle or uterus and broad ligaments.

Symptoms and Diagnosis

This abscess type presents as severe but diffuse rectal discomfort, which may be moderately exacerbated by defecation. A sense of fullness is often felt. Fever, chills, and leukocytosis frequently accompany the disease and may be helpful findings in the diagnostic process. Rectal examination reveals a fluctuating or indurated mass within the anterolateral rectal wall. In female patients rectovaginal examination is recommended to assess abscess size.

Deep Postanal / Retrorectal Abscess

A deep postanal abscess often originates from a posterior cryptoglandular infection, which leads to transsphincteric penetration into the deep postanal space. The retrorectal abscess is characterized by continuity of the cryptoglandular infection within the intersphincteric space and, by following the posterior opening of the external sphincter, invasion into the pelvis. The latter occurs very rarely.

Symptoms and Diagnosis

Symptoms are very similar to pelvirectal abscesses; in addition, pain radiates to the sacrum, coccyx, or buttocks. Rectal examination displays a protruding mass at the posterior rectum wall.

Therapy

All abscesses should be incised early and drained. Waiting for the abscess to "mature" may cause enlargement of the abscess cavity and therefore make the surgical approach more difficult; the patient suffers needlessly. The risk of incision is the subsequent development of fistula (Sect. 3.6.2). In febrile patients presenting severe infectious symptoms and those who are at increased risk (e.g., with diabetes mellitus, valvular heart disease, compromised immune system) antibiotics are suggested. Pus culture should be performed to determine the approriate antibiotic for treatment. General anesthesia is required in most patients.

In perianal and ischiorectal abscesses the incision is made at the perineum in a circular way as close as possible to the anal verge, considering the possible involvement of sphincteric muscle. A probe is inserted to assess size and continuity of the cavity. If a fistula is present, fistulotomy must be performed (see Sect. 3.6.2). After the pus is evacuated, the cavity is irrigated, and an elastic band or an iodoform gauze wick is inserted in the case of a large cavity. A light dressing is applied and the patient is dismissed with the instructions to take chamomile sitz baths, to remove the iodoform drain after 24 h and to take stool softener. Analgetics should be prescribed. If elastic bands have been inserted, the patient is seen 3 days later to remove them.

All other abscess types require transrectal drainage. It is recommended to confirm the location for drainage by needle aspiration.

The intersphincteric type is drained through the internal sphincter, removing the associated crypt-bearing area. The cut edge of the rectum and the underlying internal sphincter are sutured for hemostasis, leaving the wound open for drainage. No packing is required. The patient is instructed to take sitz baths and stool softener and is discharged.

The pelvirectal abscess is treated by placing a catheter (e.g., Pezzer, Foley, Malecot) into the cavity which is pulled out through the anal verge after 24–48 h. In women an anterior abscess should be drained through the vagina.

In deep postanal abscesses drainage is facilitated through an incision from the rectum towards the tip of the coccyx dissecting the superficial and subcutaneous external sphincter. Packing is advised and should be left for 24–48 h.

3.6.2 Anal Fistulas

An anal fistula represents an abnormal communication between two epithelial surfaces – the perianal skin and the anal canal or rectal mucosa.

The cause of anal fistulas is anal crypt infection proceeding into the anal glands and the internal anal sphincter. The acute inflammatory process of the anorectal abscess (see above) and the formation of a chronic anal fistula must be regarded as different stages of the same disease. According to the literature, approximately 20%–30% of patients who undergo drainage of an anorectal abscess show recurrent abscess formation or the development of an anal fistula. Trauma or hard stool may also lead to an interruption of the integrity of the anal canal. For further etiologic causes see Sect. 3.6.1.

Parks et al. have proposed the following classification of fistula-in-ano, depending on their topographic relationship to the external sphincter (see Figs. 35, 36):

Type I: Intersphincteric Fistula
Approximately 70% of all anal fistulas; passes through the internal sphincter, hence through the intersphincteric plane to the skin; cephalad extension may be observed.

Type II: Transsphincteric Fistula
About 23% of all anal fistulas; passes through both the internal and external sphincters before exiting through the skin.

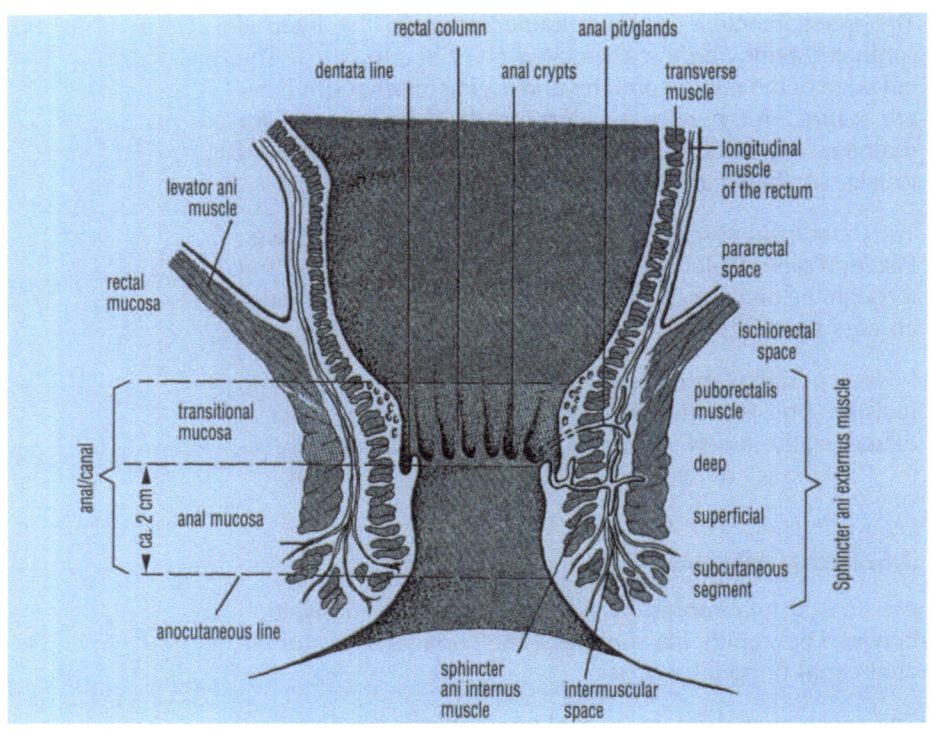

Fig. 35.
Anatomy of the
anal canal

Labels in figure:
rectal column
dentata line
anal crypts
anal pit/glands
transverse muscle
longitudinal muscle of the rectum
levator ani muscle
pararectal space
rectal mucosa
ischiorectal space
transitional mucosa
puborectalis muscle
anal/canal
ca. 2 cm
deep
anal mucosa
superficial
subcutaneous segment
Sphincter ani externus muscle
anocutaneous line
sphincter ani internus muscle
intermuscular space

Type III: Suprasphincteric Fistula

Some 5% of anal fistulas; starts in the intersphincteric plane, passing to a supralevator location, reaching the space between the puborectalis and the levator ani muscles – commonly under abscess formation – to end in the ischiorectal fossa exiting through the skin.

Type IV: Extrasphincteric Fistula

About 2% of anal fistulas; usually originates from a transsphincteric fistula (type III); passes to a supralevatoric position and to the rectum, and to the skin surface by penetrating the enire ischiorectal fossa.

In general, type I and type II fistula are treated without the risk of functional impairment of the anus or fecal incontinence. Whether or not the puborectal muscle is involved is therefore the crucial in identifying the fistula tract.

In a large series, Marks and colleagues found the internal opening of the fistula to be located in the posterior area of the anal canal in 66% and in the anterior areal in 22%. In only 12% was the internal opening found on the right or left lateral aspect of the anal canal.

A number of methods can be employed to identify the type of a fistula, the course of its tract, and the location of its internal opening; the latter includes the application of *Goodsall's rules*:

By dividing the pelvis of the patient – placed in lithotomy position – by a transverse into an anterior and posterior part, the following prognosis can be made: If the external opening lies anterior to the transverse plane and not further than 2.5 cm away from the anal verge, the internal opening tends to be located anteriorly. If the distance to the anal canal is greater than 2.5 cm, the internal opening is generally found posteriorly. Conversely, when the external opening lies posterior to the plane and as close as 2.5 cm or less to the anal verge, the internal opening is usually located in the posterior midline.

Symptoms and Diagnosis

The most frequent presenting complaints of patients with an anal fistula are swelling, pain, and discharge. The former two symptoms are usually associated with abscess; the latter implies direct discharge from the external opening. The majority of patients with a fistula have an antecedent history of abscess formation in the area.

Inspection of the anal area usually reveals the external opening as a single, pink aperture, which may close intermittently. Insertion of an olive-tipped needle opens the canal. Digital examination helps to identify the origin of the fistula: the infected crypts appear indurated, and purulent material may extrude from the crypt base. The injection of dye into the fistula tract is easy and painless: 1:2-diluted methylene blue is injected through the tract and confirms the patency of the tract and its communication with an internal opening, if it appears in the rectum. Furthermore, it makes intraoperative tracing of the fistula tract easier. It is very important not to inject the dye with too much pressure as it may then stain the entire tissue.

Identification of the complete tract in nonsuperficial fistula almost always requires general anesthesia as it causes considerable discomfort to the patient. An adequate anorectal probe is inserted and gently advanced to assess the tract's location and size. The topographic position of the fistula to the puborectal sling is determined. If there is any uncertainty concerning the position of the puborectal sling, a thick suture is placed through the tract.When the patient is alert, rectal examination is performed to assess whether sphincter contraction is localized above or below the mark.

Fistulography, the radiological delineation of a fistula tract with a water-soluble contrast agent, is helpful in patients, for example, with suspected or known Crohn's disease, detecting extensions of the fistula and possible involvement of the intestine and other organs.

Therapy

The first approach to a small, superficial fistula should be conservative, which is performed by daily irrigation of the fistula tract using saline, 1:1000 diluted povidon-iodine or 1:5 diluted TCDO. If this has no beneficial effect, surgical intervention must be planned.

Large, deep and complex fistulas almost never heal by primary intention – surgical management is mandatory.

A fistula operation should always remove the source of the disease, the anal glands and crypts. The performance of fistulotomy has proven successful in type I fistulas and in small type II fistulas, the latter with consideration of the puborectal muscle. The entire fistula tract is incised; complex fistulas may require a number of operations.

Suprasphincteric, extrasphincteric fistulas and those in aged patients with weak sphincter tonus, generally require several surgical approaches to find an individual way to maintain fecal continence. Complex fistulas such as horseshoe fistulas require unroofing and adequate drainage to the skin surface.

Postoperative care includes sufficient analgetic therapy, diet (day 1: fluids only; from day 2 on: high-fiber diet) and – very importantly – several sitz baths per day from day 2 on. The drainage tracts must be inspected daily and reopened, if necessary, to maintain exudation of material from deep spaces.

In large wounds, revision with general anesthesia is recommended on the second postoperative day. Otherwise wounds are gently rinsed, using the same agents as in

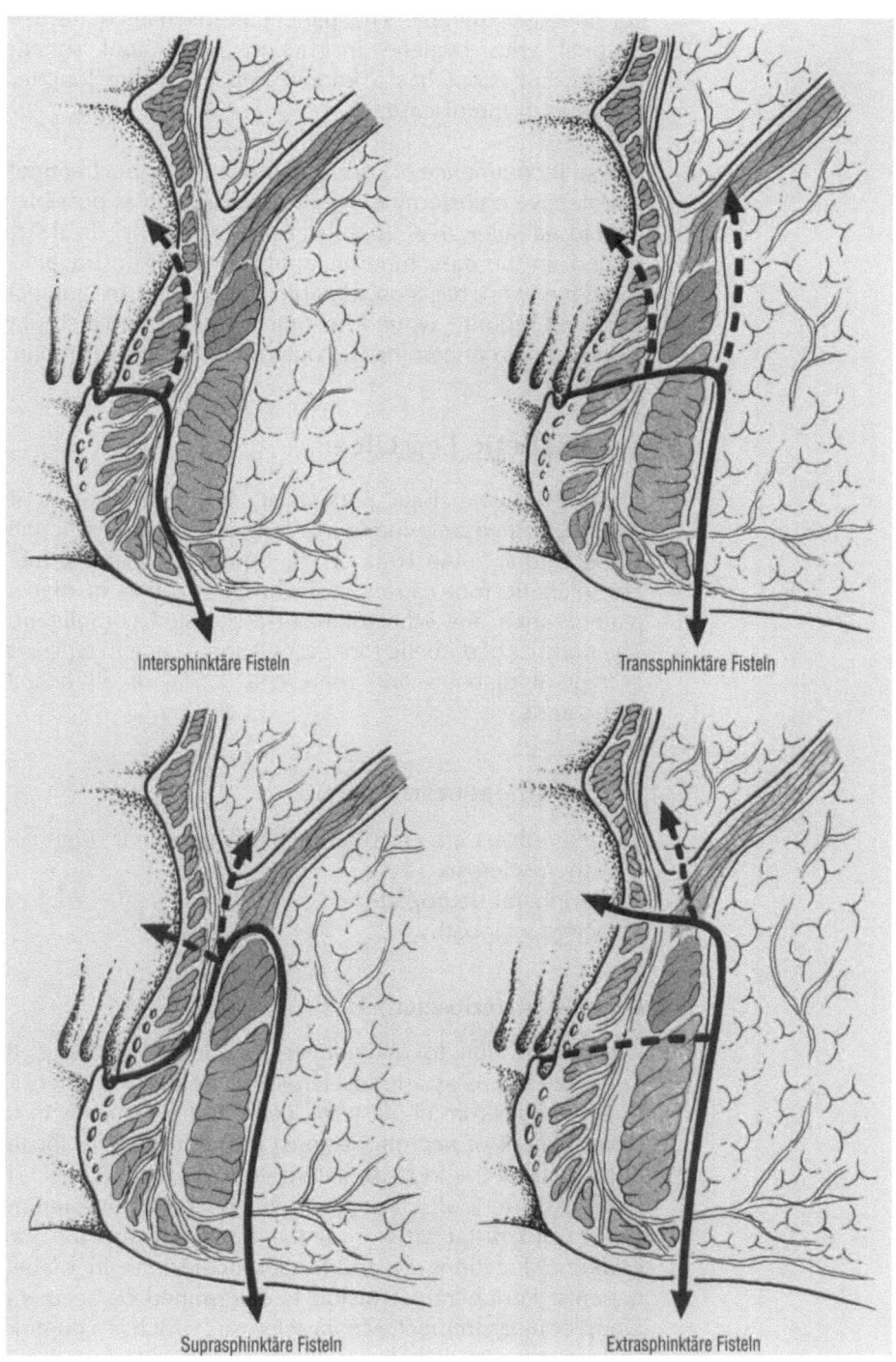

Intersphinktäre Fisteln

Transsphinktäre Fisteln

Suprasphinktäre Fisteln

Extrasphinktäre Fisteln

Fig. 36. Partially schematic representation of the major types of anal fistulas

conservative therapy. The patient is discharged from the hospital with hygiene instructions and stool softener; regular, soft stool has a known impact on the long-term outcome of the disease.

If fecal incontinence occurs after operative fistula treatment, a protective colostomy is constructed as soon as possible to be closed after 4–6 months as soon as the fistula has healed. In the meantime the sphincter is reconstructed by someone who has considerable experience in anorectal surgery. Certainly, wound healing of the excised area plays a major role concerning the outcome of sphincter repair.

3.7 Diabetic Leg Ulcer

About 25 % of diabetic patients at some point present at a specialist office suffering from a long-term complication: the diabetic foot. Some 10 %–15 % require surgical treatment. The diabetic foot causes more hospitalization of diabetic patients than any other diabetes-associated complication. The number of diabetic foot cases is increasing in type I and in type II diabetes and represents 2.5 % of all hospital admissions.

3.7.1 Pathogenesis

Diabetic ulcers are classified according to their origin:
- Atherosclerosis
- Peripheral neuropathy
- Microangiopathy

Diabetic Arteriosclerosis

Ulcerations due to diabetic arteriosclerosis produce the same symptoms as arteriosclerosis caused by hypertension or elevated serum cholesterol. Local ischemia leads to the development of necrotic lesions, characteristically located at the sole of the foot, the lateral forefoot, or the heel. The popliteal artery, distal segment of the profundus femoral artery, and distal arteries of the lower leg are the most common locations of arteriosclerotic lesions in diabetic patients. Peripheral perfusion is determined by segmental Doppler measurement. Media sclerosis, which is a common consequence of diabetes mellitus, may lead to falsely high arterial pressure because the sclerotic vessel wall appears rigid and resistant to compression. The ankle-arm index is of questionable value in these patients. It is advisable to determine the arterial pressure of each toe using a toe blood pressure cuff.

Peripheral Neuropathy

Another diabetes mellitus associated late complication is polyneuropathy causing sensory and motor impairment, paresis, and paralysis. Secondary to atrophy of the short foot muscles and the flexor muscles, toes remain in an extension position resulting in claw toes. Bony prominences of the metatarsus are pressed down causing ischemia and anoxemia. Due to the loss of pain sensation in polyneuropathy the position is not changed, but pressure ulcers and subsequent necrosis develop. Impairment of the innervation of small vessels leads to inconsistency of the capillary tonus, which also contributes to local ischemia.

Microangiopathy

A high blood glucose level has a known toxic effect on endothelial cells. Damage of the vessel wall leads to the formation of microthrombosis, obliterating arterioles, which presents as suddenly appearing areas of black infarction. The sudden insult is characteric for diabetic microangiopathy and must be differentiated from necrotizing vasculitis.

All types of wounds and ulcerations in diabetic patients are very susceptible to infection due to their impaired immune response. Erysipelas may develop from a poor wound condition.

Diabetes mellitus is strongly associated with *necrobiosis lipoidica*, which is also known as "pretibial pigmented patches;" these lesions predispose to ulceration and represent the fourth leg ulcer type in diabetes mellitus.

Clinical symptoms of neuropathy, arteriosclerosis, and microangiopathy may overlap, which requires meticulous diagnostic studies.

3.7.2 Diagnosis

Diabetes mellitus is caused by a decreased insulin production of the islets of Langerhans either by an autoimmune reaction or metabolic insufficiency in the elderly. This leads

Fig. 37.
Diabetic ulcer

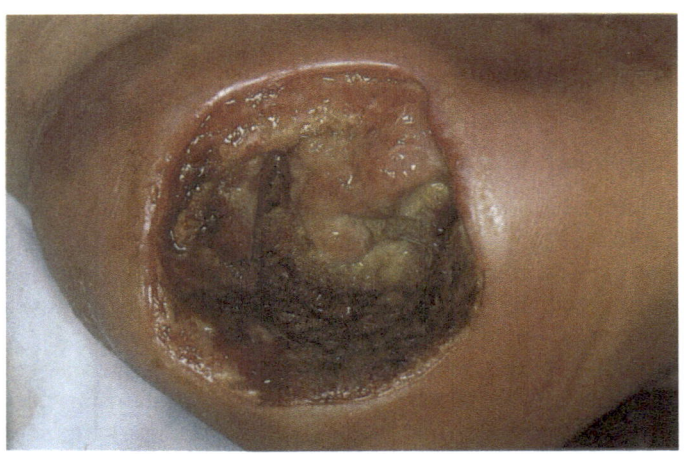

Fig. 38.
Diabetic ulcer

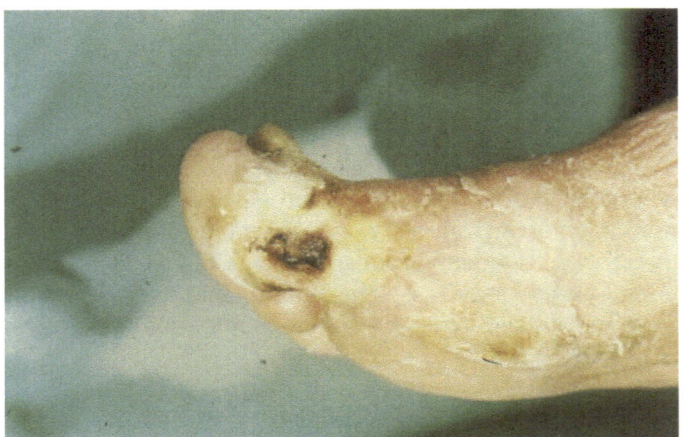

to hyperglycemia, varying between 10 and 30 mmol/l in 24 h. The blood glucose of healthy individuals is less than 5 mmol/l. This, coupled with an impaired lipid and cholesterol metabolism, contributes to media sclerosis involving arteries and arterioles. As a consequence, the hardened vessel wall is less capable of pulsation, capillary refill – determined at the toes – is retarded. As mentioned above, the ankle-arm index is often not representative because the barely compressable vessels lead to falsely high blood pressure measurements.

The first symptom of polyneuropathy is the loss of temperature perception: myelinated D-fibers and nonmyelinated C-fibers degenerate first. Early diagnosis is therefore established by performing the very sensitive temperature sensation tests. With progression of the disease, pain perception is impaired; the pen prick test is an excellent method to ascertain decreasing sensation. Nerve fibers of the sympathetic system are also destroyed, resulting in a loss of control of vasomotoractivity, loss in perspiration, and atrophy of the skin with dryness and fissuring. Sometimes the legs of diabetic patients appear reddened, which is not a sign of inflammation but of "vascular overshoot." Polyneuropathy advances from distal to proximal.

Charcot's Joints

Due to the motor impairment, examination of the toe flexors and extensors is to be very difficult (Charcot's joints). Atrophy of certain foot muscles, particularly the mm. extensores digitorum breves, may lead to the development of claw toes, hammertoes, pseudo-pes cavus, or paresis of the toe flexors. In severe cases, dangle feet are seen. In 80%–95% of these patients the achilles tendon reflex is missing. Spontaneous fractures and luxations may occur as a result of neuropathy, leading to severe disintegration of the foot skeleton. Osteolytic anomalies commonly present in diabetics and must be differentiated from osteomyelitis, which requires X-ray examination.

3.7.3 Therapy

Treatment of the diabetic foot includes modification of the insulin treatment regimens (oral antidiabetics, insulin administration) secondary to measurement of blood glucose, improvement in the patient's general condition, and antihypertensive therapy. Hyperglycemia predisposes to infection and impaired wound healing. Blood glucose concentrations within a normal range are not expected to reduce organ damage, but above all to alleviate certain types of neuropathy and microangiopathy. Improving the diabetic's general condition contributes to enhanced wound healing. This includes:

– Low-calorie diet
– Sufficient protein uptake
– Hygiene measures
– Infection prophylaxis
– Attention to foot care

Hypertension

Antihypertensive treatment is absolutely necessary to control further arteriosclerotic damage. Blood pressure must be lowered in a slow, cautious way to prevent sudden ischemia of the poorly perfused lower extremities and feet.

If closing pressure of the toe arteries is more than 60–70 mmHg, surgical débridement of devitalized tissue and amputation of some size may be performed without expecting a nonhealing wound. Additionally, the ankle-arm index (ischemia index) may be used to assess the risk of aggressive treatment: if the index is greater then 0.5, the healing rate of surgical intervention is usually expected to be more than 90%.

Infarction caused by microangiopathy is difficult to differentiate from vasculitis. Immunologically induced vasculitis can be diagnosed by positive staining for complement and immune complexes in a biopsy, obtained from a red or violet skin area.

It is not mandatory to perform cultures from chronic, unchanged ulcers; however, in an active, progressive inflammatory reaction, bacterial cultures are of crucial value.

The diabetic foot may rapidly develop progressive inflammation – erysipelas is most common – due to the ischemic condition. There is a great risk of functional loss if infection advances deep into tissue and results in osteomyelitis. Especially in recurrent, neuropathic ulcers, extended bone components and deformations should be corrected, for example, malformed heads of the metatarsal bones should be resected. Large ulcer defects require closure by surgical techniques such as skin grafts; the success of any kind of operation is directly related to sufficient perfusion of the foot, which must be enhanced by above measures. Pressure relief during the first weeks is also essential for the outcome; therefore, a plaster-of-paris is applied keeping the foot in a resting position, but allowing mobilization of the patient.

Osteomyelitis

There are two treatment regimens for osteomyelitis: surgical resection and broad spectrum antibiotics, particularly directed against gram-negative bacteria.

Topical treatment of the noninfected neuropathic ulcer includes cleaning and removal of nonviable and necrotic tissue, for example, by using proteolytic enzymes, protection against mechanic stress and relief at pressure points, such as the heads of the metatarsal bones. Occlusive dressings and the application of creams have shown no beneficial effect as they may cause wound maceration and microabscess formation with subsequent development of acute, severe infection. In terms of infection control, attempting to dry out the wounds would be the safest way; however, this has a rather nonstimulatory effect on wound healing. A commonly used drying agent is mercurous chromium solution, which has the disadvantage of staining the wound and the surrounding tissue red, masking any sign of infection. Bacteriostatic topical agents, such as carboxylic wax containing silver nitrate, sodium hypochlorite solution, or povidon-iodine, have shown good results. Note: Some agents are effective only at cytotoxic concentrations and therefore inhibit wound healing rather than enhance it.

Cave: Foot Bath

Saline foot baths and topical antibiotics are strictly contraindicated. The former tend to enhance bacterial infection.

The need for systemic antibiotic therapy is determined on the basis of clinical symptoms. In patients with chronic ulcer, there is no indication for systemic antibiotics, whereas active bacterial infection of an ulcer requires such treatment immediately. Of course, general measures such as blood glucose measurement and regulation, cleaning, and surgical débridement of the wound are performed at the same time. The choice of an antimicrobial agent depends on bacterial culture. In general, antibiotics are administered for 7–10 days. In osteomyelitis a 6-week treatment course is performed; persisting osteomyelitis patients receive antibiotic treatment for 3–6 months.

Surgical Approach

Because the vascular sympathetic tonus is usually destroyed in neuropathy, there is no indication for sympathectomy in diabetic patients. Further vasodilatation is impossible after media sclerosis. The goal of surgical therapy in the diabetic foot is arterial revascularization. Although lesions are usually located peripherally in diabetic microangiopathy, as a primary approach aortoiliac desobliteration (possibly using laser technique) or bypass is performed. This leads to increased blood flow, seen as improved arterial blood pressure measurements and a greater ankle-arm index. After arteriography similar surgical measures are undertaken at more distal vessel segments, such as at the popliteofemoral segment. Even more distal reconstructions may contribute to preservation of the foot, but these are possible only if remaining calf and foot vessels are undoubtedly intact. For imaging, puncture arteriography combined with digital subtraction angiography is the method of choice in difficult cases.

3.7.4 Rehabilitation

Preservation of the foot is not necessarily the treatment regimen of choice. Under certain conditions amputation should be taken into consideration as recovery and rehabilitation may last a markedly shorter period than with conservative measures. Early consultation of a rehabilitation specialist is therefore crucial to determine the potential goals of amputation. Amputation level, stump shape, and position of the amputation scar are planned with regard to the future prosthesis. Early exercising is essential for the patient to become accustomed to prosthesis function and to reduce hospitalization time. The latter is of extreme importance in elderly patients who tend to decompensate mentally during hospital stay.

If neuropathy is diagnosed, the patient should be advised to wear special shoes to prevent further lesions. Soles consisting of plastozot have proven successful in reducing pressure at areas of neuropathy-associated pressure accumulation, such as metatarsal bones, by dispersing it. After the sole is individually adjusted, the orthopedic shoe is manufactured by a specialist. Lightness and flexibility of the shoe are additional qualities of concern in reducing susceptibility to ulcer formation. In the beginning, perfect fitting of the shoes must be controlled monthly because the neuropathic patient does not notice discomfort produced by irregularities of the shoe.

3.7.5 Prevention

It is essential in the prevention of the diabetic foot to regularly control and, if necessary, balance the patient's blood glucose levels. General condition, weight, cigarette smoking, and blood pressure are regarded as further contributing factors and must be checked in an appropriate manner. Elderly individuals and underpriviliged persons are at special risk and must be examined with particular care by the physician. All patients are advised to check their feet and soles of their feet daily (the partner or a mirror may be of help) to detect wounds, contour changes, and diminished sensibility early on. In contrast to corns, thick callosity should be removed to prevent skin fissures. Toe nails are cut straight, avoiding sharp edges. After washing (not cold, not too hot), the feet are gently dried and rubbed with oil to avoid drying out. The patient should wear comfortable socks and shoes and should refrain from walking barefoot.

3.7.6 Organization

Optimal care is ensured whenever there is cooperation among podiatrist, nurse, physician, surgeon, rehabilitation specialist, manufacturer of orthopedic shoes, neurologist, and dermatologist. This interdisciplinary team provides knowledge and experience with the various aspects of lower leg and foot ulcers in diabetic patients, thus reducing hospitalization, frequency of amputations, expensive and time-consuming dressings and other measures, and diminishing the patient's complaints.

4 Experimental Models in Wound Healing

4.1 Cell Culture

Over the past decade the technique for fibroblast, keratinocyte, and endothelial cell cultures has improved markedly and is today relatively easy to handle. However, the extrapolation of cell culture results to the complex in vivo procedures of wound healing remains problematic.

4.2 Epidermal Wound Models

"Suction blisters" are commonly used as an epidermal wound healing model. The subbasal wound is produced by applying negative pressure to a defined skin area. The administration of cantharidin, which is the poison of the Spanish fly *Lytta vesicatoria*, leads to the formation of a suprabasal wound as it destroys the desmosomes within the prickle cell layer of the epidermis.

Additionally, the donor sites of skin grafts represent excellent wounds to investigate epidermal repair processes.

4.3 Wound Granulation Models

The experimental use of punch biopsies is a well-established model for studying wound granulation and wound contraction. Wound granulation by itself is studied by placing a Teflon ring on top of the well-prepared fascia of an laboratory animal (Fig. 39).

A major controversy in estimating the effect of pharmaceutic agents in wound healing is the objectivity of the evaluation. Results such as "good granulation" or "rapid epithelialization" are subjective categories that are inadequate for comparison to other studies. The following models have been found to be suitable for objective evaluation:

Fig. 39.
Wound granulation
model in
the guinea pig

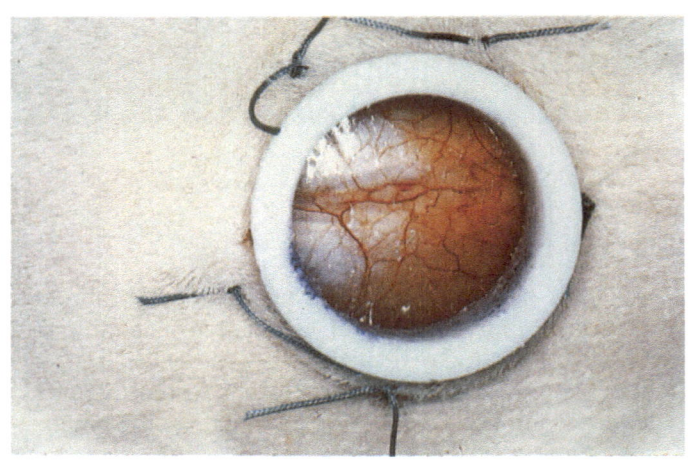

Full-Thickness Wound (Granulation Model)

The shaved back skin of anesthezised guinea pigs is used for the implantation of a Teflon ring, impeding wound contraction and epithelialization (Fig. 39). Prior to this the fascia, which forms the wound base, is covered with a polyacrylamide agar gel containing the pharmaceutic agent being investigated. The gel alone serves as control. The dressing is changed daily. Five days later the granulation tissue which has formed within the ring, including the fascia, is removed and examined histologically. The quantitative evaluation is performed micromorphometrically by dividing the specimen into ten fields of same size (Fig. 40).

Fig. 40.
Granulation tissue
layers, divided into
ten fields

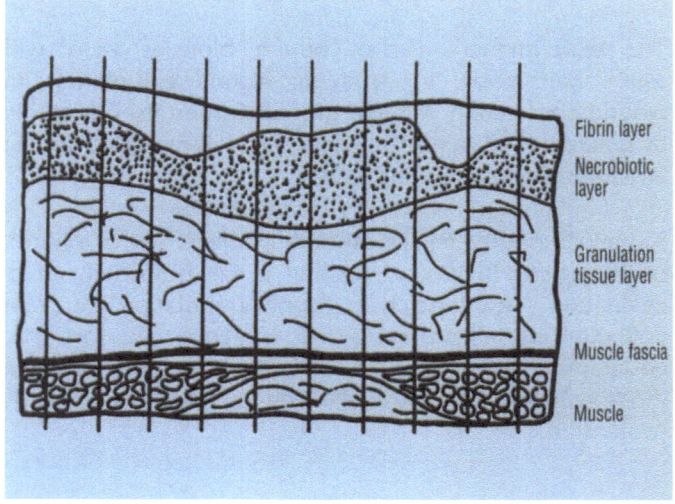

Next to each vertical line, the thickness of the granulation tissue layer, the necrosis layer and the fibrin layer is determined using a micrometer eyepiece. The mean value of ten measurements is regarded as representative for the layer size of the individual specimen (and animal); statistics are performed treating means as single values.

Full-Thickness Wound Plus Thermal Injury at the Wound Base

After the Teflon ring is implanted, the wound base is challenged by applying a temperature of 100 °C for 1 s. The further procedure is identical with the nonthermal injury wound model (see above).

Other Animal Models

Animal models resemble the human situation far more closely than in vitro models, which shorten and simplify physiological processes. The highest comparability to humans is found in the pig model due to the great similarity in skin structure. Dose-response curve studies may be performed in the pig model to find the optimal human dose.

To illustrate the use of an animal model, a study in which débridement of necrotic wounds was performed is presented below.

In Vivo Evaluation of Proteolytic Débridement: Animal Experiments

The chosen wound model should be close to reality, involving most components of homeostasis. An animal species bearing great similarity in skin structure to human skin should be selected. It is well known that removal of unviable tissue leads to enhanced wound healing. To investigate the in vivo activity of proteolytic enzymes at the necrotic wound site a randomized, double-blind, placebo-controlled study was performed in a pig model.

Necrotic ulcers were created on the back of female domestic pigs (NY) weighing 20 kg, by the following method. The epidermal and a part of the dermal layer were removed using a electrodermatome. Trichloracetic acid 20 % was applied on the wound for 4 min to cause necrosis; then the wound was vigorously irrigated using saline. The depth of necrosis was determined in four quadrants by a

Fig. 41.
Wound models

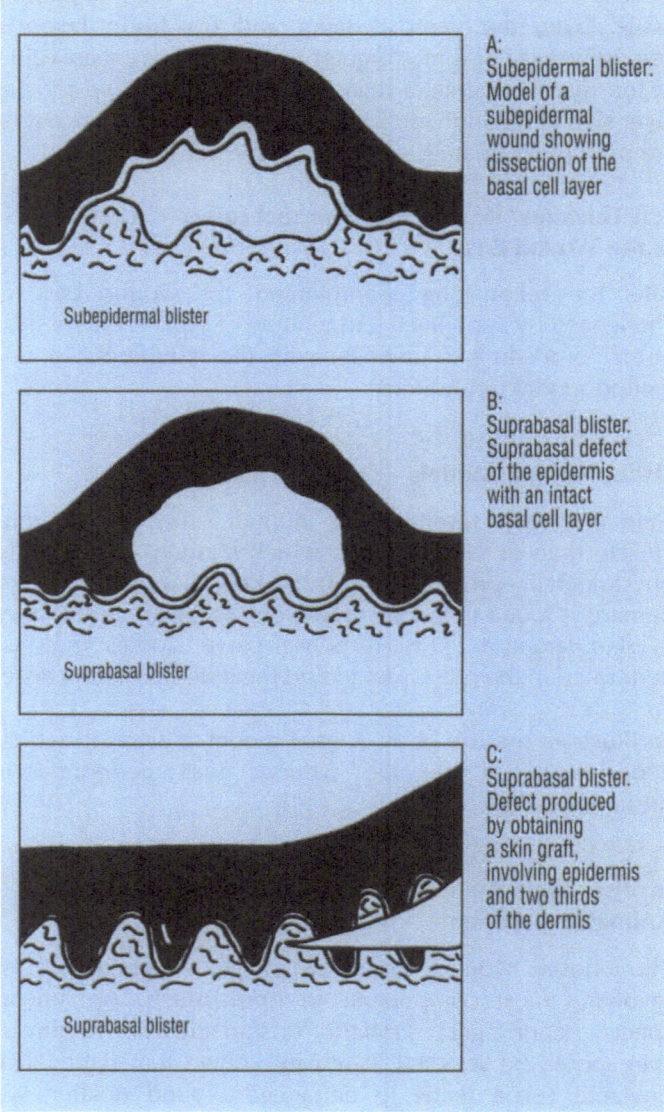

A:
Subepidermal blister:
Model of a
subepidermal
wound showing
dissection of the
basal cell layer

Subepidermal blister

B:
Suprabasal blister.
Suprabasal defect
of the epidermis
with an intact
basal cell layer

Suprabasal blister

C:
Suprabasal blister.
Defect produced
by obtaining
a skin graft,
involving epidermis
and two thirds
of the dermis

Suprabasal blister

special tissue-staining procedure (MSB staining), which marks necrotic tissue in red color and viable tissue in blue. Gauze, impregnated with five different concentrations of the proteolytic enzyme and one control, impregnated with saline, was applied on the lesion twice a day for 7 days. Wounds were controlled, measured, and photographed daily. The degradation of necrotic material was evaluated by computer analysis of the photograph. Biopsies were taken on days 4, 7, and 11 to perform routine histology, proliferation assay (bromodeoxyuridine incorporation), and cytophotometric measurement of collagen. With this animal model a valuable dose-response curve may be established, which is crucial in finding the optimal concentration for clinical use.

Subepidermal Wounds

Suction blisters are produced on the skin on the back of nude rats or at the volar side of the forearm of a test person to be subsequently unroofed. The wound is treated according to the above ("Full-Thickness Wound") cited procedure.

Until the wound is closed completely, standardized pictures are taken daily to perform planimetry; at the same time, four diameters (horizontal, vertical, two diagonal) are measured (diametry) to calculate the wound surface. The results from planimetry and diametry must correspond to one another.

Suprabasal Wounds

Suprabasal wounds are created by applying cantharidin (Fig. 42), the poison of the Spanish fly. After the blisters are unroofed, the study is carried out following the protocol of subepidermal wounds (see above).

Quantification of suprabasal wounds measures trans-epidermal water loss. The amount of water loss is directly related to the thickness of the epidermis. This is confirmed by histological examination.

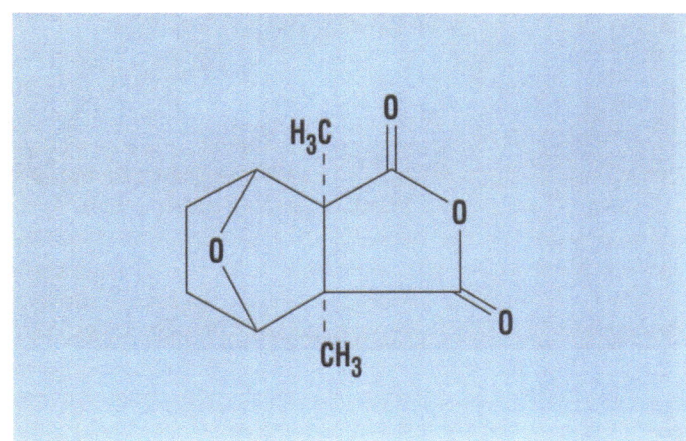

Fig. 42.
Molecular formula
of cantharidin

Fig. 43.
Nitrazin test

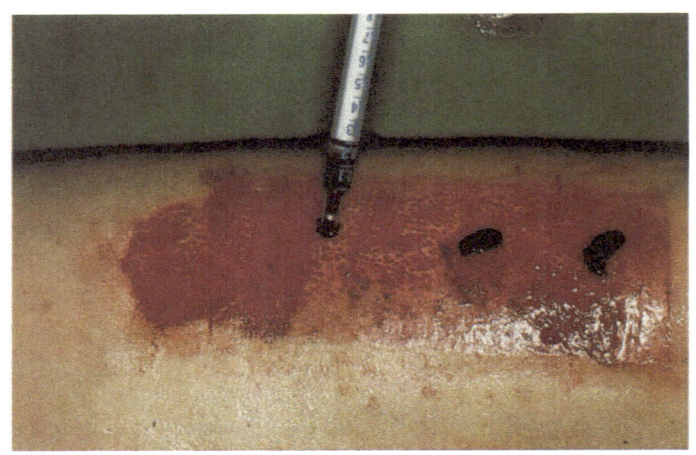

Fig. 44.
Epidermal wound

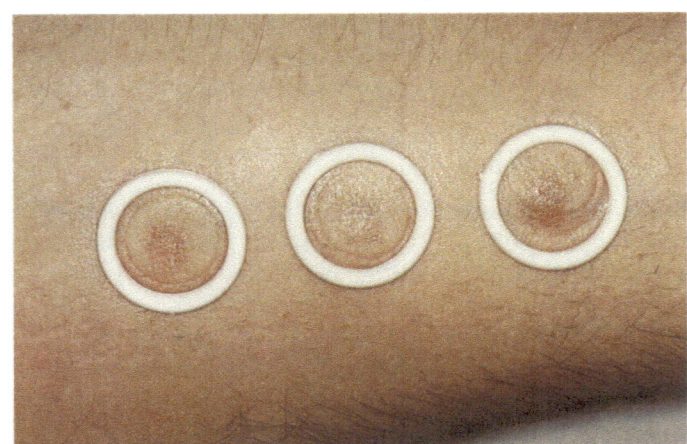

Fig. 45.
Measuring
transepidermal
water loss

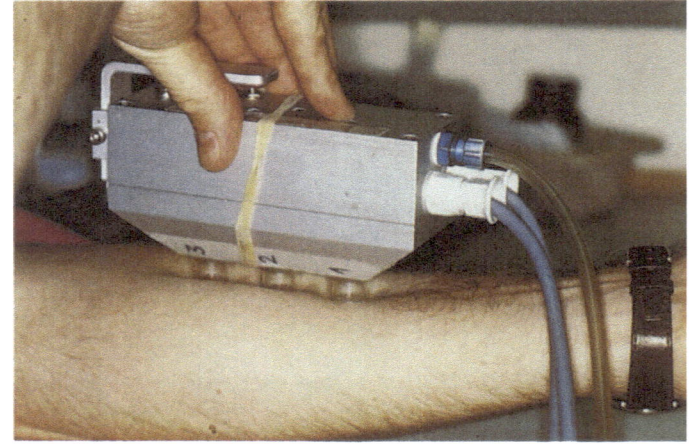

Nitrazin test: To assess reepithelialization of skin graft donor sites the nitrazin-test is used, which stains nonepitheliazed tissue blue to violet, in contrast to epithelialzed skin, which remains yellowish.

4.4 Models of Chronic Wounds

Intracorial injection of sodium tetradecylic sulfate leads to the development of poorly healing, necrotic wounds. This wound model has at least some analogy to human chronic wounds. However, there is no wound healing model for venous leg ulcer.

4.5 Methods to Examine the Progress of Wound Healing

Epidermal wound healing may be estimated by measuring transepidermal water loss, by performing the nitrazin test, by high-resolution ultrasound examination, and by testing the concentration of the key enzyme ornithine decarboxylase.

5 Topical Therapy of Chronic Wounds

Strategy of Local Treatment

Strategy of local treatment

- Removal of inhibitory factors
- Débridement
- Topical antibiotic effect
- Suppression of inflammation
- Enhancement of granulation and epithelialization
- Wound dressing

Due to the fact that wounds are of very different etiology, pathogenesis, and time course, there is no uniform therapeutic regimen. Surgical wounds heal by primary intention and require no therapy at all, besides the dressing. On the other hand, topical treatment is of major importance by secondary for wound healing.

Elimination of Local Risk Factors

Factors contributing to impaired wound healing must be eliminated or avoided. These include professional, atraumatic operative techniques resulting in a well-perfused wound area.

Accompanying illness or primary disease as well as any deficiency due to malnutrition must be treated. Furthermore, it must be considered that corticosteroids, antibiotics, antiseptics, psychopharmaceutical drugs, and antiphlogistics may have inhibitory effects on wound repair.

Local Factors Inhibiting Wound Repair

Wounds must be cleared of foreign bodies, necrosis, and hematoma; impaired circulation, germ contamination, and exsiccation of the wound must be prevented or, if necessary, treated.

5.1 Surgical Débridement

Wound Fluid Secretion Must Be Provided

The central measure in treating secondary wounds is substantial surgical wound débridement. This includes the removal of nonviable tissue, opening of wound pockets, elimination of mucous coating and foreign bodies, and the excision of infected areas. The more thoroughly a wound is débrided and cleaned, the less the risk of infection. Further, adequate drainage of wound fluid must be provided as secretory products (including blood) are an excellent medium for bacterial colonization.

Cave: Bruised Wound Margins

Areas bearing impaired blood flow, for examle, after bruising, require excision to prevent bacterial infection. Wound margins must be clean and must adapt without tension to maintain wound secretion. Skin grafting is not performed until the wound is in excellent condition.

5.2 Physical Wound Cleansing

Wet Gauze Dressing Soaked with Ringer's Solution

Wet gauze still represents a convenient and reliable wound dressing. Ringer's solution is the fluid of first choice to soak the gauze, as it contains isotonic amounts of all physiologically necessary electrolytes. Excessive use of 0.9 % saline solution leads to an electrolyte shift with subsequent retardation of the healing process.

Avoid Osmotically Active Solutions

The application of osmotically active fluids should be avoided as they may lead to wound desiccation.

Moist wound healing must be the purpose of treatment to accomplish adequate repair.

Showering and H_2O_2

Due to germ accumulation in a bath, wounds should rather be showered. H_2O_2 has excellent mechanic cleansing properties, resulting from gas formation, and is easy to handle as it is available in spray form. Its antibacterial effect should not be overemphazised.

Germ Reduction by Irradiation

Another physical method in wound healing is irradiation (UV-C). This has proven successful in reducing bacterial counts when applied daily.

5.3 Enzymatic Débridement

Enzymes play a prominent role in wound cleansing as they accelerate degradation and débridement. This results in early initiation of anabolic processes and overall enhanced wound healing.

There is a great variety of débriding enzymes and enzyme systems available which degrade different substrates (Table 5).

Indirectly and Directly Acting Enzymes

Indirectly acting enzymes must be distinguished fundamentally from directly acting enzymes. The former activate a specific enzyme within the wound fluid, in contrast to the latter, which degrade wound components themselves.

Table 5. Characterization of enzyme preparations

Name	Enzyme	Mechanism of action	Site of action	Occurrence	pH Optimum
B.subtilis protease ("sutilains ointment")	Protease	Direct	Proteins, fibrin	*B. subtilis*	6–7.5
Clostridiopeptidase A Concomitant clostridial peptidases	Collagenase Protease	Direct Direct	Collagen Polypeptides	*C.histolyticum* *C.histolyticum*	6–8
Deoxyribonuclease Plasmin (fibrinolysin)	DNase Fibrinolysin	Direct direct	Nucleoproteins Fibrin, factor I, V, VIII	Bovine pancreas Bovine plasma	7 7
Streptodornase Streptokinase	DNase Plasminogen activator	Direct Indirect	Nucleoproteins Fibrin	*S.hemolyticus* *S.hemolyticus*	7 7,4
Trypsin	Protease	Direct	Proteins, fibrin, penicillinase	Bovine pancreas	7

5.3.1 Streptokinase

Streptokinase acts indirectly by transforming plasminogen within the wound exudate into plasmin. This enzyme cleaves fibrin, fibrinogen, factor V, and factor VIII, the cleavage resulting in polypeptides and amino acids. The enzyme activator is used only in secreting wounds, as otherwise there is no plasminogen present.

5.3.2 Streptodornase

As a deoxyribonuclease, streptodornase cleaves DNA from nonviable cell nuclei into purine and pyrimidine thus liquefying viscous exudate. Viable cells remain intact. In general, streptokinase and streptodornase are applied in combination.

5.3.3 Deoxyribonuclease

The DNase is produced by bovine pancreas, cleaves nucleic substances, and therefore liquefies wound exudate. As purulent exudate contains nucleoproteins and fibrinous components at the same time, combination with fibrino-lysin is widely accepted.

5.3.4 Fibrinolysin

Fibrinolysin is a plasmin derived from bovine plasma which degrades fibrin without affecting healthy cells. In contrast to streptokinase, fibrinolysin acts directly and therefore does not depend on plasminogen containing wound exudate.

5.3.5 Trypsin

Trypsin is a proteolytic enzyme extracted from bovine pancreas. It hydrolyes ester and peptide bindings, consisting largely of lysine and arginine. Trypsin attacks denatured proteins but never affects collagen and elastin. It leads to rapid liquefaction of blood clots and incrusted exudate.

5.3.6 Collagenases

5.3.6.1 Biological Significance of Collagenases

Mammals consist up to 30% of connective tissue. Constant physiological replacement of connective tissue takes place, which requires continuous degradation and synthesis.

As extensive collagen degradation would be lethal to the organism; the triple-helical structure of collagen is susceptible to degradation by specific collagenases only. These are secreted and regulated in a very controlled way.

Collagenase Action

Collagenases degrade the substrate in a three-step process:

- Collagen fibrils are gradually attacked and softened.
- Molecules, former masked by the helical structure, are now accessible to collagenase degradation.
- Cleavage of the triple helix results in collagen fragments susceptible to other proteases.

There are two known types of collagenase: neutrophil collagenase and fibroblast collagenase. However, keratinocytes are also capable of collagenase production.

5.3.6.2 The Importance of Collagenase in Wound Healing

Breakdown of Extracellular Matrix

Polymorphonuclear granulocytes have a great capacity for infiltrating connective tissue. The breakdown of extracellular matrix during the inflammatory phase of wound healing is attributed to collagenase (metalloendoproteinase) secretion from granules of infiltrating leukocytes.

Collagen Has a Chemotactic Effect on Fibroblasts

Collagen fragments, resulting from collagenase cleavage, have been shown to act chemotactically on fibroblasts and macrophages in a dose-dependent manner.

Clostridial Collagenase Acts Chemotactically on Neutrophils

Two distinct proteases are obtained from *Clostridium histolyticum* culture: clostridiopeptidase A and neutral protease. Clostridiopeptidase A specifically cleaves collagen, thus facilitating the degradation and clearance of interfibrillar necrotic material. This bacterially produced collagenase is still the only enzyme available as a therapeutic agent which is capable of collagen degradation. Analogous to human collagenase, it is a metalloproteinase cleaving native collagen types I, II, III, IV, and V.

The second clostridially derived protease, cleaves a large spectrum of proteins nonspecifically.

5.4 Topical Antimicrobial Treatment

5.4.1 Definition of Infected Wound

Bacterial colonization of the skin is a physiological feature. A presence of pathogenic micro-organisms does not lead to infection, but is referred to as contamination.

Bacterial Counts Are Decisive

An increase in bacterial colonization leads to infection. This term is used to indicate beginning invasion of the skin or wound tissue while there may be no clinical signs of infection. With progression, bacteria penetrate viable tissue and proliferate.

From Contamination to Manifest Infection

Infection may develop from bacterial contamination whenever the following criteria are fulfilled:

- The causative organisms are contagious.
- The germs adhere to the surface and invade the wound.
- Bacteria are viable and virulent.

The affected macro-organism must:

- Be susceptible to the micro-organism.
- Show reduced immune competence or resistance.

For example, 10^4 pyogenic streptococci/mm^3 and 10^5–10^6 Staphylococcus aureus organisms/mm^3 must be present to produce wound infection. This has been confirmed in standardized experiments.

Chronic Wounds Are Never Sterile

Chronic wounds are almost always colonized with bacteria; they are never sterile. Wound contamination does not require antimicrobial treatment.

Clinical Signs of Manifest Wound Infection

Wounds must definitely be treated with antibiotics as soon as the patient shows such clinical signs as wound pain and infiltration of surrounding tissue. The wound commonly shows pus formation. Sometimes general symptoms such as fever and enlargement of local lymph nodes accompany manifest wound infection.

Complications of Manifest Infection

In most cases infection is restricted to the wound area, impairing the healing process. Theoretically any kind of infection may spread out and lead to bacteremia and subsequent septicemia, although this is seen very rarely in wound infection. Patients with lymph edema and other predisposing diseases may develop erysipelas, which is accompanied by local hyperthermia, erythema, fever, and chills.

Correct Smear Technique

Culture from wound smears very often reveals contaminating flora instead of infection-causing micro-organisms, which may be ascibed to the wrong smear technique. Smears should be obtained from the base and margins of the wound, the two locations with greatest concentration of pathogenic micro-organisms.

5.4.2 Spectrum of Pathogenic Micro-organisms

Surgical wounds and chronic wounds such as venous leg ulcer show significant differences in the prevalence of certain bacterial strains leading to infection.

Spectrum of pathogenic micro-organisms

Escherichia coli
Bacteroides spp.
Streptococcus faecalis
Staphylococcus aureus
Staphylococcus epidermidis
Pseudomonas aeruginosa
Proteus spp.
Candida albicans

Bacteria in Surgical Wounds

The most frequently found bacteria in surgical wounds are: *Escherichia coli* (18.8 %), *Bacteroides spp.* (17.4 %), *Streptococcus faecalis* (11.3 %), Staphylococcus aureus (10.5 %), *Staphylococcus epidermidis* (9.7 %), *Pseudomonas aeruginosa* (7.6 %), *Proteus spp.* (6.6 %), and *Candida albicans* (3.44 %).

Bacteria in Chronic Wounds

The leading bacterial strain in infection of chronic wounds is *S. aureus*, present in 62.9 % of cases. Gram-negative bacteria are less common (12.6 %).

Mixed Infection Is Quite Common

In 15.4 % of cases the patient shows mixed infection: culture reveals *S. aureus* in combination with gram-negative bacteria. Other studies, however, have reported in 73.1 % of infected chronic wounds gram-negative, fecal microorganisms, *S. aureus* in 21.5 %, β-hemolytic streptococci in 18.4 %, and anaerobes in 11.5 %

Fungal Infection

The most common fungal infection – present in 13 % – 39 % of chronic leg ulcer cases – is *C. albicans* infection. There is a significantly higher incidence of *C. albicans* infection in occlusive wound treatment.

Apathogenic Bacteria

Physiological skin flora. Healthy skin is characterized by a microbiotope-like colonization with certain bacteria, fungi, and protozoons. The quantity and composition change due to factors such as age, pregnancy, environment, nutrition, personal hygiene, and living conditions.

Resident flora include *S. epidermidis, S. saprophyticus, Micrococcus luteus,* Streptococcaceae, Peptococcaceae, and aerobic and anaerobic *Corynebacteria.*

Transient Flora consist of spores, gram-negative *E. coli* strains, *Actinobacter,* apathogenic microbacteria, and yeast. Viruses are not part of the physiological skin flora.

Nosocomial Bacteria

This type of infection is not dependent on the wound but on the bacterial spectrum of the individual hospital. The antiseptic hospital situation leads to the development of new bacterial genotypes, well-adapted to their surroundings, more virulent and more resistant to antibiotic therapy.

Staphylococci and Gram-Negative Bacteria in the Hospital

Staphylococci and gram-negative bacteria cause most of hospital cross-infections, far more than the former classical nosocomial bacteria streptococci and clostridia. The reason for this change is the capacity of rapid genetic transformation (spontaneous mutation) resulting in antibiotic resistance of enteric bacteria and staphylococci.

Pathogenic Bacteria

Staphylococcus aureus

S. aureus is the most virulent species of the staphylococcus genus. In culture, S. aureus forms characteristic yellow accumulations (Fig. 46b), produced by orientation changes and partially adhering cells during cell division. The diameter of the bacteria is 0.8–1.2 µm. There is no formation of spores.

Virulence Factors

The surface of some Staphylococcus species is formed by a polysaccharide capsule, which increases their virulence.

The interaction of the staphylococcal surface protein A with Fc fragments of the IgG immunoglobulin contributes to further virulence.

S. aureus produces enzymatically active toxins: coagulase, four distinct hemolysins, leukocidin, epidermolytic toxins, and enterotoxins. α-Hemolysin damages various human cells and leads to skin necrosis. β-Hemolysin, classified as sphingomyelinase C, also produces skin necrosis. γ-Hemolysin and δ-hemolysin act as surface detergents. Leukocidin attacks granulocytes and macrophages.

Staphylococcal Lyell's Syndrome

Epidermolytic toxins cleave the skin within the granular layer producing staphylococcus-associated Lyell's syndrome (or staphylococcal scalded-skin syndrome). Staphylococcal enterotoxins include staphylokinase, hyaluronidase, protease, nuclease, and lipase.

Typical Staphylococcus-Associated Infections
Abscess, furuncle, carbuncle, impetigo contagiosa, staphylococcal food poisoning, and toxic shock syndrome are characteristic staphylococcus-associated infections.

Germ Reservoir: Nose
The nose is the main bacterial reservoir. A considerable percentage (up to 40%) of infected persons present staphylococcal colonization of the nose. There is a great chance of hand contamination and subsequent transmission to the wound.

Coagulase-Negative Staphylococci
Coagulase nonproducing staphylococci, for example, coagulase-negative *S. epidermidis*, belong to the physiological skin flora. These bacteria may lead to wound infection in certain predisposed patients.

Streptococci
Streptococci are gram-positive, immobile cocci with diameter of 1 μm. There is no spore formation. The cell membrane of streptococci carries the C substance, which is a antigenic polysaccharide.

Surface M proteins are restricted to pyogenic streptococci, serological group A. These proteins are of major importance for virulence. There are now more than 70 known subtypes of the M antigen. Other streptococcus surface proteins such as T proteins, trypsin-resistant surface antigens, and the rare R proteins have no effect on virulence. The polysaccharides within the capsule seem to have antiphagocytic properties.

Three Types of Hemolyzing Streptococci
Depending on hemolysis, three types of streptococci are distinguished:

- α-Hemolytic streptococci turn hemoglobin into methemoglobin with production of H_2O_2. This reaction leads to the characteristic green dicoloration of the bacterial mass.

- β-Hemolytic streptococci degrade hemoglobin completely.

- γ-Hemolytic streptococci have no effect on hemoglobin.

Streptococcus pyogenes
Most streptococcus-associated infections in humans are produced by *S. pyogenes*, serological group A. *S. pyogenes* has the exceptional capability of spreading within tissue. Classical diseases originating from *S. pyogenes* infection are impetigo contagiosa, erysipelas, necrotizising fascitis, and scarlet fever.

M Protein Protects Against Phagocytosis
Due to the protective effect of the M protein against phagocytosis, bacteria reproduce undisturbed. The above-mentioned capability of pyogenic streptococci to disseminate within tissue is due to the production of multiple antigenic enzymes such as streptolysin O, streptolysin S, hyaluronidase, streptokinase, deoxyribonuclease (DNase), NADase, and erythrogenic toxin.

Dangerous Antibody Production
Clinical relevant streptococcal infections almost always lead to antibody production, perferably against antistreptolysin and anti-DNase B (mainly in skin and wound infections). There is an increased risk of glomerulonephritis and endocarditis 3 weeks after the skin or wound infection.

Enterococci – The Intestine as Reservoir
The intestine of humans and animals forms the physiological reservoir of *S. faecalis*. This bacterium is usually seen in combination with Enterobacteriaceae, in mixed wound infections.

Pseudomonas aeruginosa
P. aeruginosa is a gram-negative, aerobic bacterium with polar flagellae, showing catalase activity. Originally, *Pseudomonas* was known as a saprophyte, living in

rottened material of soil and on the water surface; with the development of modern hospital hygiene it became an important infection-causing agent. *Pseudomonas* infection may be easily recognized by its characteristic blue-green discoloration and its aromatic odor; therefore, it is also termed *Bacterium pyoceaneum*.

Pseudomonas – A Chromogenic Bacterium (Fig. 46a)
Pseudomonas aeruginosa produces a green fluorescing color (pyoverdin), blue-green cyanin, reddish pyorugin, and brown pyomelanin. Furthermore, it is a β-hemolytic bacterium, producing gelatinase, lecitinase, DNase, and decarboxylase.

Affinity for Large Wounds. Pseudomonadaceae show a significant affinity to large skin defects, preferably in hospitalized patients.

Clinical Features of Pseudomonas aeruginosa *Infection.* In *pseudomonas* infection wounds appear purulent, fibrinous, discharging and show ulcerations. Infection may be either restricted to the wound area or fulminantly disseminated within the entire organism.

Pseudomonas *Resides in Flower Pots.* The bacteria is found in sanitation facilities, vaporizers, incubators, respirators, hemodialysis units, and even in flower pots. Today, *Pseudomonas aeruginosa* infection is a major problem in hospital infection. Transfer occurs from one patient to another, through contaminated instruments, even via hands of medical or nursing staff.

Enterobacteriaceae
Usually enterobacteriaceae are nonpathogenic agents except, for example, in individuals receiving radiation therapy, cytostatic drugs, corticosteroids or those who are malnourished or immunodeficient due to alcoholism.

Escherichia coli
E. coli may be mobile or immobile. There are three major *E. coli* antigen types: O-antigens of the body, K-antigens of the capsula, and H-antigens of the flagellae. *E. coli* very rarely causes wound infection.

Klebsiella
Klebsiella are immobile bacteria surrounded by a capsule. It is present in the intestine of approximately 10% of the

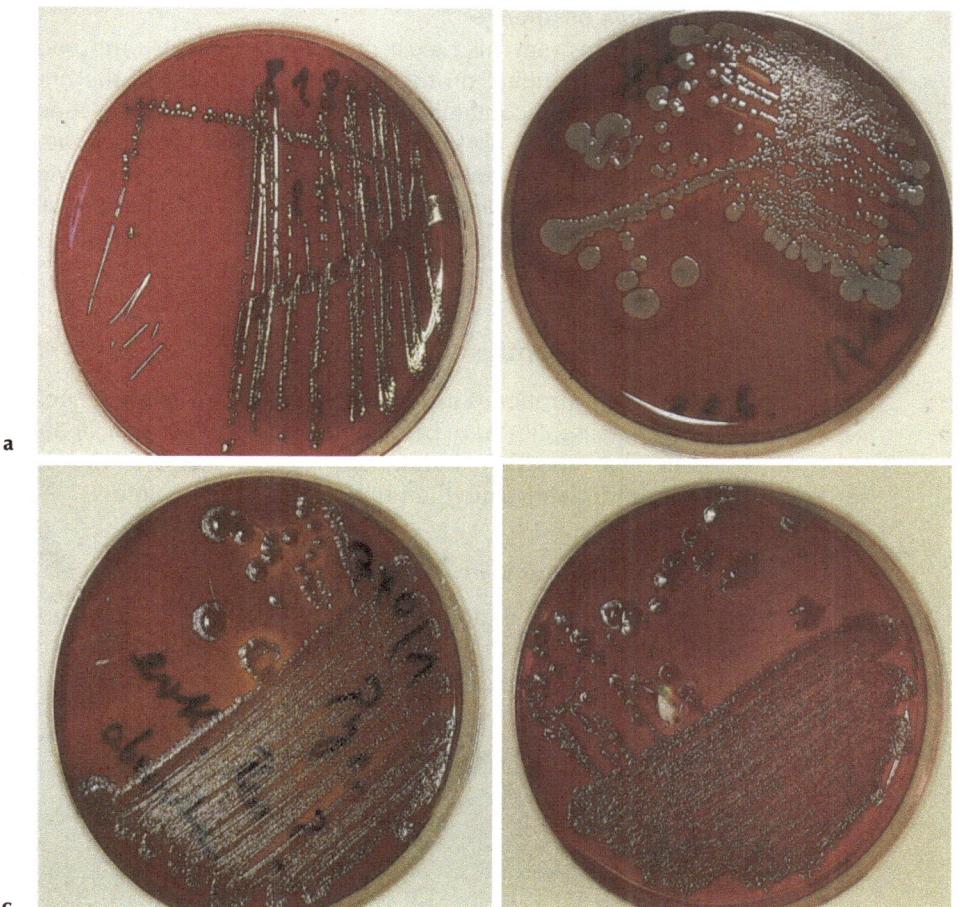

a

b

c

d

healthy human population. Typically *Klebsiella* causes pneumonia, but it may also produce wound infection.

Proteus

Since the bacterium moves spontaneously, it was termed *Proteus vulgaris*. There are more than 110 known serotypes of the infective agent typically causing urinary tract and wound infection.

Fungi on Chronic Wounds

Fungal infection of a chronic wound is almost always caused by *Candida albicans*. The *Candida* genus includes 140 species, only 10 of which are potentially pathogenic. The most prominent species is *C. albicans*, a saprophyte in the mouth (10 %), vagina (7 % – 8 %), digestive tract (15 %), and epidermis around openings of the body.

Fig. 46.
a *Pseudomonas aeruginosa* culture.
b *Staphylococcus aureus* culture.
c *Escherichia coli* culture.
d *Serratia* culture.

Candida on sponges

C. albicans may also exist on sponges, towels, and vegetables. Depending on the occlusive character of the dressing, *Candida* contamination is found in chronic wounds. For example, in up to 39% of chronic leg ulcer patients a specific *Candida* species was detected in the wound: most frequent was *C. albicans*; *C. paracrusei* and *C. tropicalis* were occasionally detected, but must be regarded as rarities.

5.4.3 Antiseptics

Since sensitization is a common side effect of antibiotic treatment, anitseptics have become more popular in topical antimicrobial therapy. Additionally, allergy seems to develop less under antiseptic than under antibiotic treatment.

Cave: Inhibition of Wound Healing

A considerable disadvantage of antiseptics is their inhibitory effect on wound healing. Table 6 summarizes negative characteristics of currently used antiseptics.

Name	Effects	Further characteristics
Ethanol Propyl alcohols	1, 2, 4	Painful; rapid onset of action at high concentrations
Iodine	1, 2, 3	Sensitization; iodine resorption must be considered; loss of efficacy in the presence of organic material
Povidon-iodine	1, 2, 4	Iodine resorption must be considered; inhibitory effect on wound healing
Phenol derivates	1, 2, 6	Resorption must be considered
Cationic compounds	1, 2, 6	Adsorption at the surface; weak antibacterial action against gram-negative bacteria
Heavy metals	5, 6	Enzyme blocking; coagulatory action
Light metals	5	Adstringent
Quinoline derivates	5, 6	
Gentian violet	5, 6	Strong inhibition of wound healing
Brillant green		Strong inhibition of wound healing
Eosin		No inhibition of wound healing

Table 6. Effects of antiseptics

1 = Bactericide; 2 = Fungicide; 3 = Virucidal; 4 = to some extent virucidal; 5 = Bacteriostatic; 6 = Fungistatic.

The almost dramatic inhibitory effect of pyoctanine (gentian violet) and brilliant green should be emphasized at this point. Eosin in contrast has no inhibitory properties and is a commonly used agent at concentrations not greater than 0.5 %.

5.4.4 Antibiotics

By definition a wound requires antimicrobial treatment as soon as wound biopsies reveal bacterial counts greater than 10^5/g tissue. This cutoff point is not absolute since the patient's condition also plays a decisive role; however, it should be considered that an increase in bacterial counts from 10^4 to 10^5 includes 90 000 germs, whereas one from 10^5 to 10^6 means 900 000 germs!

Antibiotic agents are of great importance in wound healing, applied topically as well as systemically. To influence the sequence of wound repair beneficially they should exhibit the properties listed in the following overview.

The efficacy of antibiotics is affected by several factors: although inflammation enhances the penetration of the agent, protein binding blocks its availability until all receptors are occupied. Thick-walled abscesses are almost inaccessable to antibiotics such as aminoglycosides; the latter are very susceptible to binding to pus, which considerably reduces their antibiotic activity. The acid pH within the abscess cavity leads to further inactivation of aminoglycosides.

Perfusion of the inflammatory area is increased, which results in a higher concentration of the antimicrobial agent at the site of infection, increased permeability of capillaries, and therefore enhanced penetration of the agent. Furthermore, for example, antibody and lysozyme invasion is

Advantages of topical antibiotics

Site of application = site of action
High concentration of the active substance
No systemic side effects
Antibiogram is hardly necessary
Low resorption rate

facilitated. Increased body temperature augments the action of certain antibiotics; such is seen in staphylococcus infections treated with β-lactam antibiotics.

The antagonistic effects of inflation clearly dominate over any beneficial effects. Low pH stimulates growth of many bacteria and may influence antibiotic efficacy. The action of moderate alkaline antibiotics is inhibited by the acid environment of inflammation; aminoglycosides are predominantly affected, their efficacy being markedly reduced, for example, gentamicin has a 90-fold greater effect at pH 7.8 than at pH 5.5. Chloramphenicol, clindamycin, and various β-lactam antibiotics are not inhibited by acid environment.

The presence of pus may also impair antibiotic action. Nucleic acids derived from dead leukocytes lead to complex formation with aminoglycosides. Gentamicin, colistin, and polymyxin bind reversibly to purulent cell membranes. Again, aminoglycosides are antagonized by bivalent cation (Mg^{2+}, Ca^{2+}) binding.

Necrotic material may reduce antibiotic action in terms of a diffusion barrier. Adhesion of bacteria (predominantly *Pseudomonas*, *E. coli* and *S. aureus*) to surfaces may provide protection against antibiotic action; this phenomenon is termed "surface effect" (see following section).

Antibiotics manipulate defense mechanisms of the immune system: chemotaxis, lymphocyte transformation, retarded hypersensitivity, antibody production, and phagocytosis are modified.

5.4.4.1 Bacterial Ecology

In recent years ecological aspects of bacteria have become an important topic of investigation. The term "cryptic germs" was created to describe well-hidden bacteria, hardly accessible to antibiotics. The idea of the pathogenic bacteria as the target of specific antibiotics conveniently placed within the shooting gallery has been revised. Numerous infectious diseases have been recognized to result from inaccessible foci, in which encapsulated and immobilized bacteria survive.

All bacteria may exist in two forms: either as a rather unprotected moving cell, looking for new places to colonize, very susceptible to antimicrobial attacks, or as a sessile micro-colonial form, enclosed by a mucous layer, adhering to sur-faces, surviving there even unfavorable conditions. The mucous layer, termed glycocalix, functions as a protective and adhesive factor. Therapeutic elimination of these cryptic microcolonies is quite difficult; in fact as they are very well adapted to their environment (body surface) and also reasonably resistant to defense mechanisms of the host.

As a great advantage, site of application and site of action are identical when using topical antibiotics. This leads to a high concentration of the active agent at the infection site with minimal or no systemic side effects. The great availability usually makes an antibiogram unneccessary (see following section).

5.4.4.2 Development of Resistance

Resistance is determined using the platelet resistance test. This in vitro method reveals antimicrobial action as an inhibiting areola. If the platelet has a load of 30 µg of the antibiotic being tested, and the inhibiting areola is less than 17 mm after incubation, the bacteria is categorized as "resistant" to the antibiotic agent (Fig. 47).

The clinical relevance of the platelet resistence test is of great importance whenever antibiotics are given systemically. As the concentration achieved by topical application is considerably greater, less significant resistance is seen.

However, it is well known that topical use of antibiotics triggers resistance development to a greater extent than systemic use. Resistance develops from exposure of bacteria to an inadequate concentration of the antibiotically active substance within deep tissue layers. In more detail, the surface concentration of the antibiotic is usually very high, declining with the depth of tissue; there, colonizing bacteria are not killed immediately and are therefore able to produce resistance. Thus, weakly penetrating local antibiotics bear a great risk of resistance development. On the other hand, negligible resorption is one great advantage of topical treatment in terms of systemic side effects.

To enhance the penetration rate of topically applied agents, crusted wounds must be débrided thoroughly. Débridement is of decisive character in poorly penetrating antibiotics

Fig. 47.
Inhibition areolae
produced by
antibiotic action

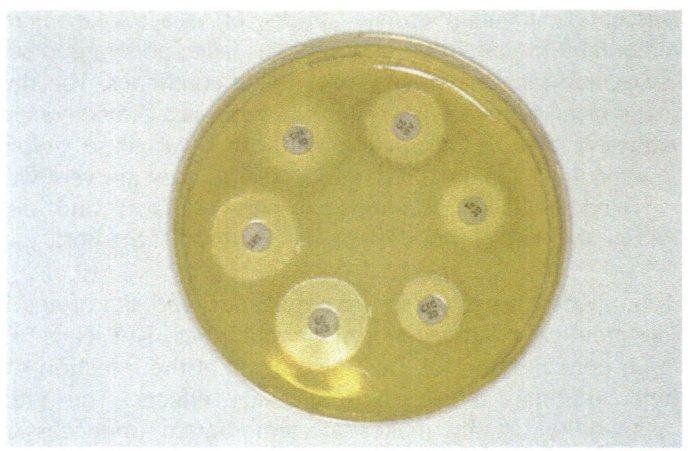

such as neomycin and gentamicin; additionally, their penetration ability depends on their galenic properties.

5.4.4.3 Allergization

A further disadvantage of the external use of antibiotics is the occurrence of contact allergies. A less allergenic agent is bacitracin. Reports on allergenic properties of the most widely used agent neomycin differ markedly depending on laboratory and patient group. An allergization rate of 3.7% was found in a selected patient group treated in European dermatological hospitals.

Sensitization obviously seems to depend on the pathological process. The external use of antibiotics on the lower

Properties required of the perfect topical antibiotic

Activity spectrum
- Specific spectrum
- Secure bactericidal effect
- Neglegible development of resistance

Physicochemical characteristics
- Stability
- No inactivation through biological material

Side effects
- No phototoxicity
- Low sensitisation rate
- No general toxicity

Local factors
- Good tissue tolerance
- No wound healing impairment

Table 7. Topical antibiotics and their effects

Agent	Combination with	Spectrum
Neomycin*	Bacitracin**	*Gram-negative bacteria **Gram-positive bacteria
Gentamicin	–	*P.aeruginosa*, Gram-negative bacteria, staphylococci
Framycetin	Enzymes	Gram-negative bacteria
Framycetin*	Gramicidin**	* and ** (see above)
Thyrothricin		Gram-positive bacteria
Thyrothricin	Neomycin	* and ** (see above)
Polymyxin B	Bacitracin Neomycin	* and ** (see above)
Fusidic acid	–	Gram-positive bacteria
Chloramphenicol		* and ** (see above)
Chloramphenicol	Enzymes	* and ** (see above)
Tetracycline	–	Gram-positive bacteria
Chlortetracycline hydrochloride	–	Gram-positive bacteria
Meclocyclin	–	Gram-positive bacteria
Mupirocin		Gram-positive bacteria

leg in diseases such as chronic venous insufficiency, stasis dermatitis, ulcer formation, and associated conditions predisposes to allergization. Apart from the pathological tissue status, long-term treatment – which is generally required – contributes to contact allergization. It is not surprising that in chronic venous insufficiency epicutaneous sensitization is found in approximately 41% of patients treated with neomycin.

A further problem is group allergenicity, which means epicutaneous sensitization against neomycin, including other chemically similar antibiotics such as kanamycin, paromomycin, gentamicin, and others. If allergy exists

Disadvantages of topical antibiotic therapy

Sensitization
Development of resistance
Insufficient penetration of the entire tissue layers
Wound healing impairment

against neomycin plus bacitracin, it is not an allergy against a group but a combination of agents, as the two antibiotics differ chemically.

5.4.4.4 Influence on Wound Proliferation

The influence of local antibiotics on wound healing should be taken into consideration. Bacitracin has no inhibitory effect on wound healing, whereas neomycin alone and the combination with bacitracin does. The least beneficial impact on wound healing is found with to tetracycline.

Even the healing process of epithelial wounds is impeded by antibiotics; therefore their use during reepithelialization should be contemplated only in serious situations.

5.5 Topical Preparations Enhancing Wound Healing

Although the elimination of pathogenic factors is the main objective in the basic therapy of deficiently healing wounds, every effort should be made at the same time to enhance the healing process. An enormous range of substances may be used, yet with varying success.

5.5.1 Electrolyte Solutions

Proliferating cells require an adequate nutrient medium. This led to the development of a solution containing the most favorable concentrations of electrolytes and amino acids. It is preferably used in burn wounds and is said to have a stimulatory effect on wound healing. In animal experiments it shows neither a stimulatory nor an inhibitory effect on the repair process of normal wounds. Maintainance of the optimal milieu is obviously not a sufficient way to enhance healing. However, in burn wounds, in a state of severe electrolyte imbalance, external replenishment of electrolyte concentrations leads to stimulation of repair.

Appropriate topical antibiotics

Bacitracin	Polymyxin
Thyrothricin	Tetracycline
Chloramphenicol	Mupirocin

5.5.2 Pantothenyl Alcohol

Pantothenyl alcohol is the alcohol of the vitamin pantothenic acid, biologically active in its dextrorotatory form. As a component of the coenzyme A, pantothenic acid represents a cofactor of certain enzymatic reactions which require transfer of acetyl groups such as gluconeogenesis, fatty acid synthesis, fatty acid degradation and synthesis of steroids, steroid hormones, and porphyrins.

Pantothenyl alcohol is well resorbed by wounds; this was shown in a trial using tritium-labeled pantothenyl alcohol. Within the organism it is transformed into the acid form.

Pantothenyl alcohol has been in use for more than three decades. So far, no objective trial has investigated its action apart from clinical case reports and from studies in which it was used as a compound of combined preparations. Both animal and human studies have found that 5 % pantothenyl alcohol enhances epithelialization. No trial has shown an inhibitory effect.

5.5.3 Tetrachlorodecaoxide (TCDO)

TCDO forms a complex with heme. Its active form resembles the peroxide-H_2O_2 complex in the presence of the halogen Cl. Presumably, oxygen is released from the TCDO complex which has a stimulatory effect on wound repair. TCDO activates wound macrophages, those playing a central role in the healing process. The presence of heme is the prerequisite for complex formation and TCDO efficacy. Furthermore, TCDO was found to have dose-dependent antiseptic properties.

5.5.4 Calcium

Calcium plays a major role in various biological processes such as enzyme regulation, release of hormones and neuro-transmitters, muscle contraction, and cell proliferation. Calcium activity within cells and cell systems is mediated and regulated by the calcium-binding protein calmodulin, which is inactive itself and is turned on by complex formation. The cytosol steady-state concentration of calcium ranges from 10^{-8} to 10^{-7} M. Concentrations of 10^{-6} M or more may be seen transiently after stimulation.

Extracellular calcium has no effect on cell proliferation as homeostasis prevents flow into the intracellular space. The combined administration with potassium leads to depolarization of the cell membrane allowing calcium to move into the cell. This enhances cell proliferation and subsequently wound repair.

A calcium-potassium preparation is indicated in all insufficiently healing wounds and in clinical studies has been shown markedly to stimulate wound granulation and epithelialization.

5.5.5 Phenytoin

Phenytoin, if administered systemically, produces gingival hyperplasia as a side effect due to its strong stimulation of fibroblast proliferation. This effect is used therapeutically in wounds and chronic leg ulcer. The mechanism of action of phenytoin is based on its influence on ion exchange: active or passive transport of sodium and calcium across the cellular or subcellular membrane is enhanced. In resting, nonexcitable tissue, sodium permeability is enhanced by phenytoin which stimulates the sodium pump; three sodium ions transfered from intracellular to extracellular are exchanged with one calcium ion transferred into the cell. In conclusion, phenytoin leads to an intracellular increase of calcium, which enhances wound granulation (see preceding section).

Several investigators have confirmed the efficacy of topically applied phenytoin. The concentration should not exceed 0.5% as greater amounts lead to a strong, cytotoxic calcium influx.

5.5.6 Zinc

Efforts have been made since the early 1960s to verify the stimulatory effect of zinc on wound healing. The results are conflicting. Systemical zinc administration shows a beneficial effect on wound healing only in zinc-deficient patients. No change in wound repair is seen when nondeficient indivduals receive zinc supplementation.

The topical application of zinc results in a high, pharmacologically active concentration. The increase in wound granulation is due to the fact that zinc is an essential part of several enzymes, thus activating DNA and RNA synthesis. Secondly, zinc inhibits the enzyme dipeptidyl-aminopeptidase-4, which reduces fibrin aggregation; therefore the construction of the fibrin net is improved. Further, anticoagulatory enzymes are inhibited by zinc: urokinase, plasminogen activator, and α_2-macroglobulin. It is not yet understood how zinc affects the inhibition of calmodulin-dependent processes, for example, Ca^{2+}-calmodulin-ATPase, as calcium stimulates DNA synthesis and fibroblast proliferation, as mentioned above. Although the molecular pharmacology of zinc is not yet fully understood, its main action seems to be the triggering of RNA and DNA synthesis, subsequently activating collagen metabolism, and enhancement of fibrinogenesis, which in turn is augmented by fibronectin. Fibronectin forms the matrix of granulation tissue and is of great importance in terms of collagen formation and maturation during the reparative phase of wound repair.

Clinical trials have shown that zinc ions augment proliferation processes in wound healing, however, restricted to wound granulation. Epithelialization appears to be rather suppressed with zinc therapy, which emphazises its effect on fibroblast activity.

Topical preparations enhancing wound healing

Electrolyte solutions	Sugar
Pantothenyl alcohol	Dextranomer
TCDO	Cadexomer
Calcium	Heparin
Phenytoin	Hirudin
Zinc	H_2O_2
Silver nitrate	Potassium permanganate
Silver sulfadiazine	Ketanserine
Aluminum	Inosine
Chamomile	Allantoin
Chlorophyll	Vitamin A
Refined mineral oils	

5.5.7 Silver Nitrate

The application of silver nitrate leads to protein precipitation due to silver ions reacting with sulf-hydryl-, carboxyl-, and amino-groups. This explains the partially adstringent and antimicrobial effects of the agent. Bacterial suspensions are killed, even at a concentration of 20 ppm in distilled water, which is term an oligodynamic effect.

Silver nitrate is used preferably as a therapeutical agent in chronic leg ulcer at a 0.2–1 % concentration. Experimental studies have shown that administration of 1 % silver nitrate leads to a slight inhibition of wound healing. The use of 2 % silver nitrate reduces wound secretion, destroying newly formed epithelium. At a concentration of 0.5 % does silver nitrate did not impair epithelialization of burn wounds but of the donor sites used for skin grafting.

At a concentration of 0.2 %-silver nitrate is definitely non-toxic in terms of wound repair. It shows antiseptic activity against both gram-negative and, to a lesser extent, gram-positive bacteria. In vitro a 0.0039 % concentration is sufficient to kill *S. aureus*, and a 0.000013 % concentration to kill *P. aeruginosa*. This data is not quite transferable to the in vivo situation, since a concentration of 0.2 % is required to obtain bacteriostatic activity.

5.5.8 Silver Sulfadiazine

Silver sulfadiazine is used extensively as a topical burn care agent and in infected wounds. Its antimicrobial activity is explained by dissociation of sulfadiazine (damage of the bacterial wall, interference with folic acid synthesis) and silver (damage of the bacterial cytoplasmic membrane). As the preparation has a preferential activity against *pseudomonas*, it is commonly used in infected leg ulcers and those which start to scar. Silver sulfadiazine is barely resorbed; therefore it is well tolerated. Side effects such as exanthema, and maceration of surrounding skin are seen very rarely. The use of silver sulfadiazine is strongly contraindicated in pregnancy, sulfonamide allergy, and glucose-6-phosphate dehydrogenase deficiency.

5.5.9 Aluminum

Aluminum forms complexes with higher molecular weight substances exhibiting antiphlogistic activity. Application forms for therapeutic use are aluminum powder, foil, or coated cellulose. Its precipitating and antiedema activity are experimentally verified.

5.5.10 Calf Hemodialysate

Various animal experimental studies have revealed that application of calf hemodialysate on wounds leads to increased disruption strength on postoperative days 5–9. Hemodialysate treatment of open wounds in pigs and guinea pigs enhanced granulation tissue formation and vascularization. Its stabilizing effect on the cell membrane is controversial.

5.5.11 Chamomile

Chamomile gauze has antiphlogistic activity. Its use is indicated in wounds at the exsudative stage of repair in which the moist gauze significantly enhances the pharmacological effect of chamomile.

5.5.12 Chlorophyll

Chlorophyll-containing preparations are generally oxidizing agents. They are used in fetid wounds, their odor handicapping the patient's social contacts.

5.5.13 Refined Mineral Oil

Therapeutic agents containing mineral oil locally induce a local inflammatory reaction which is believed to restart retarded repair processes.

5.5.14 Sugar

Granulated sugar topically applied leads to a decrease in swelling due to its hyperosmolar effect. Fibrinous and putrid chronic wounds or wounds healing by secondary intention are candidates for sugar therapy. Some patients may experience granulated sugar therapy as painful or unpleasant.

5.5.15 Dextranomer

Dextranomer contains dry, hydrophilic beads which consist of branchless dextran chains linked to each other by glycerin in a chemically stable way. The linkage is performed in three planes resulting in a three-dimensional network. Dextranomer properties are wound fluid uptake and removal of necrotic wound material and bacteria. This cleans the wound. Due to the finding that dextranomer-treated wounds show an increased number of cells and an enrichment of ground substance, patential stimulatory effects of dextranomer on granulation tissue formation and vascularization have been considered.

The network of hydrophilic macromolecules is capable of absorbing great amounts of fluid such as serum and pus, but also eliminates nonviable tissue, inflammatory mediators and, micro-organisms. It is an effective agent only on exsudative or purulent ulcers or similar discharging lesions. Dextranomer is an inert substance without any serious side effects. High costs are the limiting factor of usage.

The microbeads are applied directly on the wound, covered with an occlusive dressing for 24 h. With every dressing change the wound must be rinsed with saline to remove the used beads. Its use in paste form is more convenient to apply. The cleaned ulcer is covered with a moist, sterile gauze on which dextranomer paste is spread out; this is followed by an occlusive dressing. The procedure is repeated every 24 h until an almost dry, granulating wound base results.

Displeasing side effects include pain due to the osmotic effect (as with sugar) and dessication of the wound.

Dextranomer is employed mainly in chronic wounds such as leg ulcer and decubitus ulcer and polyvalently sensitized patients, because no contact allergies have yet been reported.

5.5.16 Cadexomer

Cadexomer-iodine is a hydrophilic three-dimensional network consisting of a modified starch polymer. The matrix incorporates iodine at 0.9 %. Cadexomer has adsorbing activity; at contact with wound exsudate it swells to form a gel, which slowly releases iodine. Due to the antiseptic effect of iodine, cadexomer is indicated in chronic wounds presenting bacterial superinfection.

5.5.17 Heparin

The anticoagulatory effect of heparin is used topically in wound healing to eliminate microthrombi, which appear physiologically following to local hypofibrinolysis at wound edges, or to prevent their formation. It is not yet confirmed whether heparin enhances tissue fibrinolysis. However, mucopolysaccharides such as heparin do have a stimulatory effect on collagen biosynthesis of fibroblasts.

When heparin is applied on a fresh, open wound, the fibrinolytic activity leads to bleeding. Alopecia is a very rarely seen side effect of topically applied heparin.

5.5.18 Hirudin

The goal of hirudin therapy is prevention and removal of microthrombi within the wound area, which are seen, for example, in one-third of chronic crural ulcers. As in all agents enhancing fibrinolysis, there is a risk of bleeding when hirudin is applied on fresh wounds.

5.5.19 Hydrogen Peroxide

The release of oxygen atoms from hydrogen peroxide (H_2O_2) creates a short-term desinfecting effect. The high concentration of catalase in purulent wounds leads to an enormous release of oxygen, visible as vesication. This process results in mechanical cleansing – a far more important effect than the weak antiseptic activity.

Purulent, fibrinous wounds are candidates for hydrogen peroxide treatment, which may be accompanied by an unpleasant burning sensation within the wound area. It should be used with caution as wound margins may be irritated toxically. Contact allergies have not yet been reported.

5.5.20 Potassium Permanganate

Potassium permanganate has oxydizing, deodorizing, antiseptic, and fungicide activity. In a concentration range of 1:2000–1:5000 most bacteria are killed within 1 h. It should be noted that the presence of organic material markedly reduces the antiseptic effect of the agent. Potassium permanganate is preferably applied on excessively discharging wounds in (moist) gauze form.

5.5.21 Ketanserin

Ketanserin is a serotonin antagonist which is used systemically in arterial hypertension and peripheral arteriopathies. When applied topically as an 2% ketanserin creme, it enhances microcirculation (inhibition of platelet aggregation, reduction of capillary permeability) and stimulates granulation tissue formation (angioneogenesis, acceleration of collagen synthesis and cell division). These effects have been confirmed in double-blind studies. Ketanserin is a well-tolerated, promising agent, which will be of great use in the future.

5.5.22 Inosine

As an endogenous physiological nucleoside, inosine plays an important role in chemical reactions supplying the human metabolism with energy. Exogenously applied, inosine is rapidly resorbed due to its excellent membrane penetration. It represents a basic component of adenosine and xanthosine monophosphate (purine) synthesis, which in turn is required for the composition of nucleic acids. Inosine is also transformed into phosphoribosyl pyrophosphate, essential in combination with nicotinic acid for NADP synthesis. In the literature inosine is reported to have beneficial effects on granulation tissue formation and epithelialization. However, until now only few studies and no double-blind trials have been performed.

5.5.23 Allantoin

Allantoin is either produced synthetically or extracted from the plant *Symphytum officinale*. It has been in use for a long time in the treatment of crural ulcer. The urea compound acts keratolytic whereas the hydantoin moiety has antiphlogistic and anesthezising properties. According to recent investigations, epithelialization is stimulated by allantoin.

5.5.24 Vitamin A

Vitamin A plays a major role in inducing and controlling epithelial differentiation and proliferation processes by effecting an increase in mitosis rate and cell metabolism. In vivo and in vitro studies in animals and humans have confirmed its stimulatory effect on cell proliferation. Conflicting results have been published concerning its impact on fibroblasts; however, its beneficial influence on

therapy increases wound disruption strength.

Critical Remarks

Except for certain calcium and zinc preparations, our own studies have shown no measurable wound healing enhancing effects of most of the presented agents. However, inhibitory effects were rarely seen; therefore there is no contraindication for their use in clinical practice. Published clinical trials generally reveal subjective observations which are hardly testable by objective criteria.

Experience, for example, in ulcer therapy shows that any preparation initially shows great efficacy, but that this subsides after some time. If a second agent is then used, healing is promoted. Therefore, dynamic therapeutic concepts should be emphasized in chronic wound treatment.

The objective in optimal wound healing is not to disturb the course of repair but to avoid impairing effects in order to prevent retardation of the healing process. Sufficiently healing wounds are most probably not susceptible to stimulation by any agent. In general, the main objective of wound treatment must be elimination or minimization of inhibitory effects.

6 Wound Dressings

The choice of wound dressing represents a fundamental decision in therapy. Dressings have distinct granulation- and epithelialization-affecting qualities. Occasionally, negative effects (e.g., bacterial growth) must be contemplated in selecting the right dressing. The great advantage of modern wound dressings is the maintainance of moist wound conditions in contrast to the "classical" gauze technique, which leads to the formation of a dry, firmly adhering coat that is even resistant to enzymatic débridement. Furthermore, there is a marked water loss associated with temperature decrease, which retards biochemical processes of repair.

The Objective of Moist Wound Treatment

The main objective of moist wound treatment is to imitate the condition of an intact wound blister. The humid milieu has a stimulatory effect on cell proliferation and migration of epithelial cells. The goal of wound dressings was to formerly protect the wound from secondary infection by forming a barrier against bacteria and absorbing wound fluid.

Occlusive Wound Treatment

There are three categories of occlusive wound treatment devices: semipermeable films, semiocclusive hydrogels, and occlusive hydrogels.

6.1 Semipermeable Dressings

By definition semipermeable dressings are permeable to steam, oxygen, and other gases. Water and bacteria cannot permeate. Steam permeability is 2500 $g/m^2/24$ h. Non-covered, granulating wounds have a steam loss of 5000–7000 $g/m^2/24$ h. Thereby semipermeable dressings prevent wound dehydration. Gases in molecular form diffuse the membrane and dissolve in the wound fluid. The O_2 permeability of certain products ranges from 4000 to

$10\,000$ cm³/m²/24 h. Usually semipermeable dressings are made from polyurethane, one side of it coated with adhesive material.

Composition of Semipermeable Dressings

Transparent polyurethane foil
Absorbing membrane made from polyurethane
Porous adhesive layer: atonic acryl adhesive

Indications: Crural ulcer, decubitus ulcer, first- and second-degree burns, abrasion and lacerated wounds, skin transplants.

Contraindications: Deep wounds with muscle, uncovered tendons or bone, vasculitis, systemic infection, arterial ischemia.

6.2 Hydrogel Dressings

A major disadvantage of semipermeable dressings is the large accumulation of wound fluid, which is not absorbed. Hydrogel dressings, in contrast, have a great capacity of fluid absorption due to their structure: three-dimensional networks of hydrophilic polymers made from gelatin, polysaccharides, polyelectrolyte complexes, and methacryl ester polymers. They swell with the uptake of water until an equilibrium is accomplished, thus collecting a considerable amount of wound fluid.

6.3 Hydrocolloid Dressings

The combination of polymeric hydrogels with elastomeric and adhesive compounds is termed hydrocolloids. Elastomers as well as adhesives are produced from synthetic hypoallergenic material. Hydrophobic layers contain hydrophilic particles. The most common gel substance in hydrocolloids is carboxymethylcellulose, which firmly adheres to the wound margins after contact with transepidermal water. The hydrocolloid part, overlaying the wound, swells to 12 times its weight by absorbing fluid.

Isolated gel islets become confluent. This process is termed phase reversion: by fluid uptake, the initially hydrophobic component turns hydrophilic. Phase reversion is clinically apparent as cushion formation, which implicates a marked decrease in adhesiveness. The dressing may then be removed in an atraumatic manner.

Alginates

Alginates are produced from alginic acid, which is extracted from brown algae (*Laminaria* spp.) and processed into calcium alginate. In contact with wound exsudate, unsoluble calcium alginate turns into soluble sodium alginate through ion exchange. This initiates swelling associated with a great fluid absorption capacity. Single gel fibers may remain on the wound throughout dressing changes and dissolve within the exsudate. There is no need of mechanical elimination of these particles since they are washed away with time.

Odor Absorbing Dressings

The fetid odor of chronic wounds may markedly influence the social contacts of the patient. Considering this, the patient should be treated with odor-absorbing dressings.

Swelling Capacity

Hydrogels and hydrocolloids swell in the presence of fluid. Their capacity of water uptake is quite limited since hydrogels already consist up to 95% of water. The quotient calculated from the initial volume and the volume after 24 h contact with fluid is termed swelling index. Hydrocolloids swell in a linear way and have a great fluid absorption capacity. The more exsudate present, the more the gel extends into the wound. This has a secondary beneficial effect: pressure is applied on the wound, which enhances granulation tissue formation. Furthermore, the colloidal gel presents an absorption gradient for soluble substances of the wound exsudate thus eliminating toxic compounds of bacteria and cell debris. Those hydrocolloids containing proteins and polysaccharides may interact with cells, effecting wound healing by releasing monomers. This may be the first step from reactive to interactive wound therapy.

Effects of Occlusive Wound Treatment

– Enhancement of epithelialization (e.g., freshly incised wound: about 40 %)
– Stimulatory effect on granulation tissue formation and on recovery of chronic wounds (acceleration of dermal fibroblasts migration and collagen sysnthesis)

Disadvantages of Occlusive Wound Treatment

Promotion of Wound Infection

Wound dressings should be chosen according to the stage of repair. If there is strong wound exsudation, any type of occlusive dressing must be avoided since fluid accumulation makes the wound very susceptible to infection, and subsequent impairment of the healing process may occur. In these wounds, absorbing nonocclusive dressings must be used.

The use of sterile gauze has not proven successful since it leads to rapid development of unsterile wound conditions by absorbing fluid and blood. Secondly, when the dressing dries, it becomes rigid, and unflexible and adheres to the wound, which makes dressing changes extremely painful. When drainage is maintained, nonadhesive foils may be applied to the wound.

Preferably, polyurethane foam should be used in granulating – especially prior to grafting – rather than in epithelializing wounds. In some case this measure is disadvantegeous because newly formed sprouts may be ripped off during dressing changes.

Much is demanded of the ideal wound dressing (see below). The use of the dressings presented in this chapter assures moist wound healing, which is the optimal condition for reepithelialization. Furthermore, they stabilize epithelial migration.

Ideal properties of a wound dressing

Adequate fluid drainage
Absorption of wound fluid
Permeability for gas
Moist wound condition
No release of fibers or foreign material
Nonallergenic and nonirritating
No adhesion to the wound base
Protection against contamination
Easy to handle
Painless dressing changes

7 Growth Factors – A Future Prospect?

The family of growth factors includes:

– Epidermal growth factor
– Transforming growth factor
– Fibroblast growth factor
– Nerve growth factor
– Platelet derived growth factor

Wound healing is regulated by a very complex interaction of growth factors. These in turn are controlled by the extracellular matrix. The use of single growth factors in the therapy of insufficiently healing wounds has not lived up to its expectations. A future concept may be a growth factor "cocktail," consisting of various factor at certain concentrations. Moreover, the expression of growth factor receptors under wound healing conditions is still a matter of investigation. Experimental trials must also rule out possible risks such as oncogenic effects of growth factors.

Subject Index

Italic numbers refer to figures

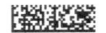